Where Did My Wife Go?

Understanding And Surviving Menopause,
Mid-life Crises
and the Empty Nest Syndrome

Jim Vigue

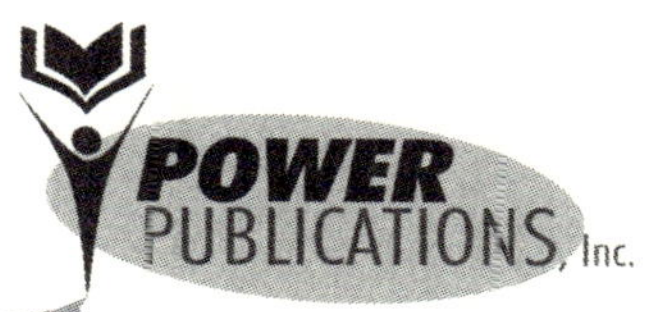

This book contains advice and information relating to health care. It is not intended to replace medical advice and should be used to supplement rather than replace regular care by your doctor. Seek your physician's advice before beginning any medical program or treatment. The publisher and the author disclaim liability for any psychological or medical outcomes that may occur as a result of following any of the suggestions in this book.

Published by Power Publications, Inc. Printed in the United States of America. The views expressed or implied in this work do not necessarily reflect the views of the publisher or the printer.

ISBN 978-0-9724194-8-2

Table of Contents:

Introduction:

This is my fourth book. In the past I've written on such diverse topics as investments and baseball. If you had told me 24 months ago I would be writing a book concerning these subjects of menopause, mid life crises and the empty nest syndrome, I would have thought you were nuts. Actually if I hadn't experienced this myself I wouldn't have believed it. After two years of personal experience and much research, I am willing to admit that an understanding of the subjects discussed in this book is vitally important to every couple in America.

With the huge financial meltdown we are now experiencing, the mood in this country as I write this book is not great. Every day we see media stories regarding the frailty of the economy and plunging real estate values. People are worried and scared. As hundreds and hundreds of billions of dollars of home equity disintegrates with falling real estate prices across the country you have to ask yourself if anyone really cares about declining hormone levels.

Fortunately, eventually markets do turn but hormone levels usually don't unless you do something about them.

The truth of the matter is that people do care. They understand that there is a problem but they just don't know where to turn to get help. That's why early last year I decided to change the focus of the foundation that I established over 18 years ago. Based on experiences I had gone through I was determined to help other men understand and deal with these complex issues that confront middle-aged women. The fact is that too few women get help in these areas (especially from their OBGYNs), and if they don't understand the problem or how to deal with it, what chance do their spouses have of understanding them?

I also feel that there is now a growing awareness of how hormones affect lives in this country. One is the way they affect relationships and the other is the way hormones affect health. In the December 2007 issue of *Life Extension* magazine the cover story was about how hormones are taking the place of drugs in fighting killer diseases. When you think about it, that certainly makes perfect sense. As we age and get older our hormone levels start falling and that's one of the main reasons that we are susceptible to the diseases related with aging. If we could maintain those youthful levels of hormones into our 50s, 60s and 70s, perhaps we could ward off a number of these diseases. There is a great deal of scientific data that appears to back this up.

So the fact that hormones could influence our health caught my attention and then when I personally experienced that hormones can also affect other areas of life besides health, I decided to spread the word.

What I have learned from personal experience is that hormones are very powerful and can change a person literally overnight. Unbalanced hormones affect the circuitry of the brain in a way that can change personalities. And when personalities can change, lives can also change. In my case it was one minor operation that dramatically altered the hormones of the woman I loved. In reality it threw a seemingly healthy woman into an instant artificial menopause. The way she explained the feeling was, "Something just snapped. In one day I felt completely different about you. It was like a light switch to our relationship had been shut off."

During my research I have learned that many women (and men) *can* deal with the conditions of menopause over an extended period of time. But if it is immediately thrust upon them, it's more difficult to deal with. Some women are thrown into it and have to deal with everything at once. That is what happened to my wife. One day after her operation she was a different person and our 25-year relationship was changed forever.

This book is about trying to understand what happens when women go through menopause and the various additional life-changing events of both midlife crises and the empty nest syndrome. Unfortunately I had to deal with all three at the same time.

If I hadn't been in love with my wife, this all could have been much easier to accept and deal with, but I still loved her, making the pain of the experience even more pronounced and difficult to understand.

The reason I am writing this book is perhaps to help a few men understand what is going on and what they might be able to do to be able to get through it. (Frankly there were days when I didn't think I could get through it).

Hopefully this book will give you some ideas that you may be able to use to prevent some of the negative events that ultimately take place in most long term relationships. Perhaps some ideas and strategies will help you to be better able to deal with these events and finally, if all else fails, maybe it will give you some steps you can take to move on with your life and find happiness again with someone else.

There are many things in life over which we have no control, and having spouses fall out of love with us is certainly one of them. It's something none of us wants to go through but many of us do.

If the material in this book can help keep just one marriage and one family together, I will consider it a great success.

PART ONE
UNDERSTANDING

ONE:

Man To Man

An E-Mail To Jim

Hi, Jim…

It was great meeting you on the court yesterday. You played a good game and gave me a real workout and I needed it. I just wish we'd had the time to talk more before I had to get to my meeting. I really need to talk to someone about what's happening. So I hope you don't mind if I unload on you. Here goes.

Right now I feel like everything in my personal life has come to a screeching halt. Things are not good between my wife and me and it tears me up so that I can hardly concentrate on my work. It didn't get this bad overnight, of course. But I had made excuses for months before it all came to a head due to a frayed electrical cable.

The electrician's report wasn't good. He said the ancient cable in the 100-year-old house we had purchased wasn't up to code and the wiring had to be replaced everywhere. The main service was only 60 amps and needed to be upgraded to 100 amps to handle the new kitchen we wanted to install. Even without the added energy drain from the new appliances, the current load being consumed was far greater than the current wiring could handle since it was probably between 40 and 50 years old and the rubber casing itself had deteriorated. Nothing was grounded, there were bare wires all over the place, and we had frequent shorts and mini-brownouts. The house was actually in danger of burning down. It was an accident waiting to happen, and we needed to take care of the situation immediately. No question. We had to do something right away to avoid disaster. So we hired a professional to rewire the entire house. Several months and several thousand dollars later, the new wiring was working great. But the marriage was in worse shape than ever.

Looking back on the rewiring experience, it was very similar to what happened to my wife, Cheryl. We had been happily married for 22 years (or so I thought), and then during the course of a year she morphed into someone I didn't recognize and decided she really wasn't interested in married life anymore (including sex) and just wanted to be free to do her own thing. She'd taken care of the home, the children, and had helped me in my business all those years and she'd just plain had enough, announcing, "It's time for me to do what I want for a change." Then she added,

"By myself." My heart hit bottom. It felt as if it had actually stopped beating.

I was shocked at the direction our marriage was taking to say the least. I had actually been looking forward to this time when the kids would be on their own and Cheryl and I could move to a less frantic schedule and rediscover ourselves as a couple. But it appeared that was not going to happen.

All through the rewiring mess Cheryl had not been feeling great—bleeding 25 days out of 30 every month, irritable, with a lot of pain and cramping. We knew she had several fibroid tumors in her uterus and it seemed to me that it was time to do something about it. But every time we talked about it, she wanted to put it off. She became more and more withdrawn and communicated less and less. Obviously sex was the last thing on her mind. I understood, but I missed the intimacy.

After several months of this I convinced her to see a new doctor. She had mentioned an operation she had read about that was supposed to be minimally invasive and had been successful in destroying fibroids without having a hysterectomy. Cheryl had heard so many horror stories about hysterectomies from her friends that she didn't even want to talk about that option. She went to see the doctor and decided to have the ablation, a process that flooded the uterus with a solution that supposedly destroyed the fibroids so that they would shrink and eventually flush themselves out of the body.

The operation went well, but it didn't work. I didn't know it at the time, but Cheryl would never be the same. She began bleeding again, heavier than before. Our relationship took a steep nosedive. Basically what happened is that the operation caused an artificial menopause. She was 45 at the time, so we had been expecting natural menopause to hit soon. (The dreaded M-word!) But I don't think either one of us expected the complete destruction the artificial menopause brought to our marriage. One day Cheryl was the same loving mother and wife I had lived with for over 20 years and the next day she was someone I no longer recognized. Mood swings, loss of concentration, biting remarks designed to hurt not just me but our three children, too, became the norm around the house. She was obviously through with nurturing.

In the bedroom it was worse. It wasn't just the desire for intimacy that was gone. She didn't even want a hug from me. No physical contact whatsoever of any kind at any time was the new rule. We slept in the same bed, but if we accidentally bumped against each other, we apologized and moved apart.

The change was so sudden it was mind-blowing. I found myself having an identity crisis of my own. I remembered and focused on the good things we had shared and the life we had enjoyed together. My wife, however, only focused on the not-so-good things that had happened to us and magnified it all way out of proportion to what had actually happened. If this was my new wife, what did that make me, and where did our relationship stand? How was I supposed to deal with my own still strong love for her and my physical needs and, even worse, the loss of the best friend I'd ever had?

I began doing research online and located medical people in our area who practiced natural approaches to menopause. After multiple visits to multiple OBGYNs, naturopaths, and other medical practitioners, Cheryl had endured many tests and had tried many types of treatments but she continued to suffer incessant periods and mood swings that surprised even her. She freely admitted she felt awful 99% of the time and didn't know what to do about it.

Eventually all the doctors were telling us the same thing: The unending bleeding had caused her to be anemic and she needed a complete hysterectomy. Nothing else had worked. This was the only option left.

The hysterectomy was successful and Cheryl recovered—physically. I have to admit that things are better around the house, but they are not even remotely approaching good. There is still no intimacy, and no communication on the deep level we had before our lives fell apart. It's as if her brain and emotions have been completely rewired—just like our house.

Last week Cheryl told me she thought we had no chance of getting off the emotional and physical roller coaster until we negotiated a trial separation. And that's where we are now. Maybe then we'd have a shot at getting back together and moving on. I still love my wife and I want her back. But I'm at a loss to know how to achieve that. Can we get back to what we had before? Will it ever be the same again? Is there something I can do? If you have any suggestions, I am anxious to talk with you.

Thanks, Jim, for listening. See you on the court?

Ted

Hello, Ted…

It was good to hear from you, although I was saddened to read what you've been dealing with. Believe me when I tell you that you are not the only man I know who is going through this hard time in his marriage.

Several of my friends have shared similar stories with me, but that is only the tip of the iceberg. This is what can happen with menopause. It rewires a woman's brain so she only sees the bad stuff *and* she magnifies it way out of proportion to what it actually was at the time. This is a key. In all likelihood your wife is likely only thinking about those bad times and has magnified them by 1000 percent in her own mind.

One of my friends wrote me a note very similar to yours. He said, "During that terrible year I devoured every book from every angle imaginable that I could find on the subject of menopause. I read over fifty books and learned a great deal. (One thing I learned was that there are few, if any, books written for men whose wives are going through this.) Bottom line: Menopause had rewired my wife's brain so that she literally was not the same person I had married and lived with for over 20 years."

If you're reading this and nodding your head in agreement, I want to give you the help you need in understanding what's happening to your marriage. I did some research and learned that there is help available, but it's not that easy to find. So I've pulled some resources and information together for you (and several of my other friends who are in the same boat as you). The following pages should help you through this tough time in your marriage, and give you some options.

If you have questions or just want to talk, call me. I'm with you in this, Ted. There *are* things you can do to help your wife through this difficult time and it *is* possible to save your marriage. Divorce is *not* the answer. Call me anytime you want to talk.

How about 10 A.M. on Friday for tennis? I'll reserve the court.

Jim

TWO:

What Happened To Her?

"I'm such an unholy mess of a girl."
Kathryn Hepburn
The Philadelphia Story 1940

Some women sail through menopause without even noticing it. (They might be in the minority.) Some women go through a readjustment of their physical lives and come out the other side with a renewed zest for life and a new freedom to explore their own sexuality and deepen the marriage relationship. Some women, however, suffer such a total change—both physically and emotionally—that they simply give up on the old life (and marriage) and go off on their own to start over in a different place with a new lifestyle and, sometimes, with a new man.

There are things you can do to turn the situation around. (And, yes, you can be the only one trying to save the relationship, but more on that in chapter five.) When it comes to menopause, first you need to really understand the problem. Men need to understand that the tried and true rule that there is a cause for every effect is not necessarily true during menopause. This is not a situation that can be analyzed, dealt with, and then it goes away. It's complicated.

In 1850 life expectancy was 38 years. Now it's more than double that. Most women back then didn't live long enough to experience menopause. Back in 1850 gynecology and obstetrics were just a part of every physician's practice. It wasn't until recently that insurance companies would even allow an OBGYN to be designated as a woman's primary doctor. That backward thinking has kept women from discovering what was happening to their bodies and their psyches as a result of the changes they were experiencing before, during and after menopause.

The menopause years extend from the years prior to the actual cessation of monthly periods (called peri-menopause) to the adjustment years after the periods completely disappear. When a woman has not had a period for an entire year, she is considered post-menopausal. Perimenopause can last up to ten years, but it's usually shorter than that, and is a time marked by various physical signs signifying that changes are coming, such as hot flashes and menstrual irregularity.

Women's bodies begin to change as early as the late 30s. Hormone levels drop, affecting their moods, body shape, and sexual desires. For example if a woman's estrogen level is more dominant due to dropping levels of its balancing hormone, progesterone, the result can be fibroid tumors and heavy bleeding during monthly periods. When it gets to this point, unless a woman is getting help in balancing her hormones, sometimes the only cure is a hysterectomy to remove the uterus and often the ovaries as well.

If nothing is done to regulate the hormonal levels, the woman will experience full-blown menopause with all its consequences—some good, some not good. One of the most misunderstood—and least expected—consequences of menopause is how all this change affects the brain. The parts of the brain most likely to be affected are the areas that store and process memories that are painful to the individual woman, and consequently, feelings of anger and sadness occur more frequently and are in the forefront of the menopausal woman's mind. She may cry much of the time for no apparent reason. She may be so angry she loses control. Or she may change from a reasonable person to one who seems totally out of it, exhibiting behavior that seems totally out of character for her.

Another contributing factor to a woman's sense of malaise is what has been called the empty nest syndrome. This usually occurs during a woman's mid-to-late forties when the children to whom she has devoted twenty years of her life are ready to step out on their own as young adults. Suddenly they don't need her anymore. Like airplanes lined up for takeoff on a runway, they leave home one by one and fly off to explore the world and their new-found freedom. The coincidence of the children's leaving and the woman's entry into menopause can so totally upset the marriage and the home-life that the husband is left behind in the dust, shaking his head in disbelief and confusion. It's a very scary time for everyone.

This is also the time when a woman may take a long, hard look at herself in the mirror and a magnifying glass and wonder who is looking back at her. The law of gravity has kicked in when she wasn't looking and she sees saddlebags on her upper thighs, drooping breasts, and enough wrinkles to rival a prune. In her mind her beauty has gone forever and she sees herself as totally unattractive. That's when the fear of aging hits her full force. (It's often the time when bottle after bottle of anti-wrinkle cream begin to resemble soldiers in a row on the bedroom dresser or on the shelf in the bathroom.) Not only does she not recognize herself physically but she also doesn't know what she's supposed to be doing now that the children are on their own. Suddenly here she is with herself— a situation she has not experienced before. (She's not really alone because her husband is right there, ready to enjoy the next stage of their married life. But she *feels* alone.) But the fact that she now has time for herself makes nurturing *herself* a primary focus. Actually women need to take care of themselves first so they can be better nurturers throughout the child-rearing years and through menopause. Remember the airline personnel telling the adults to put on their own drop-down oxygen masks first so they can take care of the children who are traveling with them? It's the same principle.

Nurturing herself is a good thing (and should have been happening all along), but, unfortunately during menopause, nurturing her marriage is of much less importance to her. Part of that is because she now has the time and the excuse to take care of herself instead of others. Her reasoning is that she has taken care of the children, the home, and the husband for whatever amount of years and now it's her turn. She has her own permission to do exactly that. She is at a strategic crossroads in her life; however, with the changes in hormonal levels, she is nowhere near prepared to cope with it.

One of the saddest aspects of this entire scenario is that the hormonal imbalances have resulted in her total inability to reason her way through the quagmire of shifting physical, mental and emotional changes to realize what has happened and do something about getting back to who she was before.

About 5,000 women enter menopause each day. If a woman's primary physician doesn't prepare her for the fast-approaching changes of the menopause years, the underlying issues may not ever be dealt with and menopause becomes just something the woman simply has to endure and survive however she can. Often a stronger birth control pill, vitamin supplements or an antidepressant are prescribed and that's as far as some doctors go. Most women are able to gradually work through the physical side of menopause. Some, however, experience such daunting emotional and mental issues that their brains actually function differently than they did before all the changes hit them. An accurate description is that, for these women, the brain actually is rewired through the menopause process.

How, exactly, does this rewiring happen? Hormones coordinate and influence the body's functions and can change a person's behavior. Different cells have receptors for the different chemical messengers called hormones. Any given cell in the body will be responsive only to the hormone for which it has receptors. For example, one hormone, oxytocin, is known as the touch hormone because it makes people less anxious and, in women especially, it brings out their nurturing side. Studies have shown that people who claim to be falling in love have high levels of oxytocin in their blood. It's easy to assume that if a woman's hormones are out of balance (particularly oxytocin), her nurturing nature is also out of balance.

The problem is that during the menopause years a woman's hormones are all over the place. Beginning with perimenopause, both the pituitary gland (the part of the brain that produces a sense of calm and serenity) and the parts of the brain that handle painful memories and feelings of sadness and anger (the hypothalamus), are all being constantly over-stimulated by hormonal changes. Particularly for the woman enduring menopause, both the hypothalamus (handling pain, anger and sadness) and the pituitary (handling calm, serenity and emotional peace) glands are continually bombarded. It's enough to drive even the calmest person crazy! She is in emotional over-drive—a state of being that can literally wear her out if it continues too long.

This emotional upheaval is happening continuously for the menopausal woman and affects every single aspect of her body, mind, and spirit. If there are unresolved conflicts or people in a woman's life that she has not forgiven for whatever reason, this is the time all those memories surface from the subconscious into the conscious. It's no surprise that what goes on in the mind directly affects the body. What men need to do is recognize that (particularly during menopause) what a woman goes through in her body has a very direct and noticeable effect on her mind.

One area of change that is very noticeable during the hormonal shifts of menopause is a decline in a woman's libido. This is often an area where men have a very difficult time understanding what is happening to their relationship. The trouble is that for women, sex begins in the mind. Surveys have shown that about 50 percent of the women participants reported a drop in their sex drive during menopause. The decrease was not usually a permanent shut-down of the libido, but temporary, brought on by hot flashes or fatigue. A woman's sexual drive is not always affected by menopause, but her sexual organs are always affected. Because every woman is different, so is every menopause, so it's important not to put everyone in the same box and expect the same symptoms.

While all this is going on with the women, their male partners usually don't have a clue what is happening. When the man is puzzled by what he sees as bizarre behavior, all he knows is that his woman is so unlike what he's used to that she seems like a totally different person. He begins to ask himself, "Where did my wife go?" Sometimes the women ask themselves the same thing. It's a very challenging and confusing time for everyone involved, children included. It's a sad and staggering statistic that the second-highest divorce rate in America is for couples who have been together over 25 years. After living together that long, one would hope all the kinks would be worked out of the relationship. Then along comes menopause and there is an entirely new set of kinks to deal with—and no operator's manual to explain how to do it.

If this is the situation a man finds himself in when menopause hits his wife like a bulldozer, what is he to do? Some men make an initial effort to understand and adjust, but give up too soon, divorcing their wives or moving on to another partner. Some grudgingly accept the changes in their partners and learn to live with the revised version of their mates, convincing themselves that living together as housemates with no sexual intimacy is okay. Others become proactive and take steps to help the women through the process. And even if the men do everything possible, sometimes it still doesn't work out the way they want it to.

That's why it's very important for men suffering through menopause with their wives to take care of themselves as well as help their wives through this transition.

Actually midlife and menopause are opportunities for both women and their spouses to enter a more relaxed and fulfilling stage of marriage. It's a time for them to grow their minds, hearts and souls and develop their uniqueness to make this stage of their lives a time of contributing to the lives of those around them as well as a time to explore gifts they may have been too busy to exercise previously. Husbands can help their wives have a positive attitude by having positive attitudes themselves. Men need to realize that the woman's aversion to sex is probably not due to anything they did, or to them personally. It's just biology. Affirming the woman's beauty and inner value should assure her that you do not see this as a negative change. It's simply a shift of focus. Menopause is a phase of life, not a death sentence.

Menopause has so many faces that it is easy to blame it for every problem in a marriage. Your wife may just be exhausted. She may not be sleeping well due to being wakened by hot flashes complete with soaked sheets and nightgown. Women also feel everything more deeply during this time, so be aware that an explosion of pent-up emotion is not necessarily due to something you did. It may just be something she cannot hold in any longer.

Most menopausal women crave understanding from their husbands during these upsetting times. Of course no man can fully understand the complications of menopause on an experiential level, but he can certainly understand that his wife is in an emotional and physical upheaval. If understanding and patience came in pill form, every man with a menopausal wife should take one of each every day. Both women and men living through menopause feel off-balance and totally overwhelmed, wondering if their marriages will survive the forces trying to pull it apart. Here, at last, is something a man can do when his wife is experiencing a debilitating sense of being overwhelmed: Help her out. Take over some of the daily chores around the house. Cook dinner. Take the trash out without being asked. Do it without expecting a thank-you. She will appreciate your efforts, even if she says nothing.

In addition to all the internal and emotional changes a woman's body endures during menopause, there is also the outward appearance to deal with as her body ages (seemingly before her eyes). Wrinkles, skin that resembles crepe paper, sags, bags and droops everywhere no one wants them—it's adding insult to injury. Losing her youthful image makes some women insecure. Anything you can do to reassure her that she is still beautiful to you will help her cope with the moods of menopause.

If a woman has primarily defined herself as a mother for 20 years or more, another dimension is added to the mix. If she has been the perfect example of traditional motherhood, she will be feeling a huge sense of loss of identity when the children leave home. And, due to the cessation of periods, she probably won't ever be pregnant again. Many women are so focused on the changes that age brings that they are programming themselves to ignore the accomplished and interesting person they have become over the years. Small wonder that women have such mixed feelings and need all the emotional support their men can give them.

Because women are individuals, they react differently to menopause. The only thing some women do with menopause is go through it. Others look forward to their new freedom and new beginnings in their lives after menopause. Middle-age and the menopause years can usher in a fulfilling and exciting time in a woman's life. But to get to that point, both the woman and her man have to get through the hormonal shifts of menopause.

Keys To Understanding

• *If a woman's primary physician doesn't prepare her for the fast approaching changes of the menopausal years, the underlying issues may not ever be addressed. She will simply endure and survive the best way she can.*

• *What a woman goes through in her body has a very direct and noticeable effect on her mind.*

• *Because every woman is different, so is every menopause, so it's important to not put everyone in the same box and expect the same symptoms.*

• *Don't give up too soon on your marriage.*

• *Take care of yourself so you can help your wife through this.*

THREE:

Not Tonight, Honey

"It's Hard to believe that you haven't had sex for two hundred years."
"Two hundred and four if you count my marriage."
Diane Keaton and Woody Allen
Sleeper 1973

There is no question about it: It still takes two to tango, but what does one partner do if the other one simply doesn't feel like dancing? The fact is that women need an emotional connection to enjoy sex and men need sex to have an emotional connection. Men have more testosterone than women, so, for the most part they have a higher sex drive than women. This is an age-old problem that has confronted the sexes throughout history.

When a woman's hormone levels are unbalanced, it is not uncommon for her to lose her interest in sex and to see a significant drop in her libido. While this isn't always the case, it is very common. Most men will say they don't get enough sex and most women will say they couldn't care less. This often leads to major problems with the relationship.

There is one study that reports that 86% of women suffer some drop in libido during peri-menopause or menopause. This could be loss of desire, vaginal dryness, painful intercourse or a basic loss of sensation. If 86% of women are reporting a problem with their sex drive it isn't too much of a leap to figure out that 86% of their husbands are probably suffering as well.

Men need sex to feel wanted and needed. They need sex to feel loved. Women for the most part believe that when men want sex, they are simply seeking the physical release of orgasm. This simply isn't true and often leads to significant disagreements and misunderstandings within their relationship.

Sexual desire is very complicated and, while it is easy to place most of the blame on the wild hormonal swings of menopause, there are also other factors that come into play such as a basic dissatisfaction with the relationship itself. It is a proven fact that when couples resolve some of their relationship problems, their sex life improves. So while a lower than normal testosterone rate might be a contributor it isn't the *only* contributor to lack of sexual desire in women. For some women the sex drive is simply placed on hold while they navigate the major life changes that are brought on by these hormonal shifts. However, this holding pattern doesn't have to become a permanent part of their lives.

The way a woman responds to her husband is based on many factors. Some of these factors can be emotional, others can be physical or psychological and even some financial. But a central problem is that husbands don't understand the needs of their wives and wives don't understand the needs of their husbands. If they did understand these needs, there would be a lot fewer broken marriages. It's a matter of viewing the issue through a different perspective.

Some studies have shown that sex isn't more than a 15% contributor to satisfaction in a good relationship but an 85% contributor to dissatisfaction when the relationship is going poorly. A good sex life probably means that other positive things are happening with the relationship and a bad sex life could mean there are significant problems with the relationship.

Most women want their husbands to be good providers, good husbands, good fathers *and* monogamous. But women often withhold sex if they aren't in the mood. This can cause a lot of resentment and anger in the relationship because men can't identify with this viewpoint. There is usually no problem if both parties *can* do without sex but if one party desires it and the other doesn't oblige in some way, it can become almost an unbearable situation.

Adding menopause to the mix only magnifies the problem. When a woman's hormones are unbalanced, she often isn't interested in sex or in men in general. It may not be a personal thing with her husband. She just may not want *any* man to invade her space when she is going through the hormonal upheaval. Unfortunately it is too easy for the husband to see this rejection as very personal and very damaging to his sense of self esteem.

There are things a woman can do to help the marital relationship survive menopause. Having a hormonal checkup is one of them. Having a simple blood, urine or saliva test could uncover deficiencies in certain hormones. A low testosterone level could be the major cause of the problem.

Women who are going through menopause may find their libidos in hibernation while most of their husbands will find their libidos definitely *not* hibernating. When a woman is going through menopause, most of the normal arguments just won't work. If she expects her husband to be faithful to her, then she probably shouldn't withhold sex, but in actuality she probably has no interest and couldn't care less.

It's important to note that good sex isn't about unusual positions or where you are when it happens. Good sex is about emotional intimacy, as well as physical intimacy. For women intimacy begins in the mind and manifests itself in the physical aspects. For men it's usually the other way around.

When women go through menopause that part of their brain that houses bad memories is activated and enhanced by hormonal changes. (See chapter two.) Holding a grudge doesn't work in the sex department. In fact sex does help you forget (at least temporarily anyway) by releasing oxytocin in the body. When a woman is having an orgasm, the part of her brain that governs fear and anxiety and, to a certain extent, stress, is switched off. So while she may not feel like having sex, once she gets into it, it is probably very helpful to her. She should not do it just to please her husband; she should do it for herself as well.

Sexual activity has many benefits. Depression (or a depressed mood) is often a factor in menopause, but sex reduces depression. Orgasm releases endorphins and benefits a person as much as a five-mile run. Sex also boosts estrogen levels which help reduce certain negative effects of menopause. Sex is an excellent relaxant and often better than a drug. It boosts the immune system. More sex boosts estrogen levels and that is good for the bones and helps prevent osteoporosis. Sex brings partners closer. It's something special that you don't share with your friends. It's the element of passion that makes your relationship special. There are, of course, lots of additional plusses but the chances are good that your wife probably doesn't want to hear them. That being the case what is a man supposed to do?

Perhaps the better question is: What should the woman do?

If she doesn't care about her marital relationship she can do nothing. She can simply withhold sex. There is nothing more ego-deflating to a man than to know that his wife does not desire him. This will cause him to clam up, shut down, feel rejected and perhaps even lash out at his wife. If there is no physical intimacy, the relationship has a slim chance of surviving.

If, however, the wife is aware of her hormonal issues and is trying to do something about them (seek proper medical care, for instance, from someone who is experienced in natural hormone replacement), then there are things she can do.

She can simply do it. If her husband wants sex then she should be prepared to have sex even if she isn't in the mood for it. Sometimes once the foreplay starts, a woman's mood can change quickly. It's the mental resistance that is more powerful than anything. If a wife tells herself her mood isn't right, or she doesn't find her husband attractive (another sign of hormonal upheaval), she can always lack interest. Sometimes the Nike slogan is the best motivator: *Just do it!* This solves lots of problems. Anxiety levels will drop dramatically because the shame of withholding sex is gone as is the fear of being deprived of it.

If a weak libido is the case in your marriage, consider doing something sensual with your wife, instead of something sexual. Sensual activities foster a sense of safety and well-being and togetherness. Examples would be walking on the beach, cuddling in front of the fireplace, giving each other a backrub—anything involving the senses but stopping short of having sex. Sensual activities can lead to sex, but if they do not, don't hold it against your partner.

At menopause all those hormones that used to foster the nurturing part of a woman's nature seem to be missing. A woman's perception of her life often changes as do her emotions and overall outlook on life. After a lifetime of caring for others she begins to think more about herself and her needs. If a woman finds that she isn't exactly thrilled with the way her life has turned out it is not uncommon to see a reduced libido as a result. Sometimes if a husband doesn't understand these changes, he can do irreparable damage to the relationship. This is a time for new beginnings and new ways of doing things if there is going to be any hope of rekindling the passions of a couple's early relationship.

A hormonal imbalance can often be addressed with proper medical care or the addition of natural hormones or nutritional supplements. But if she is dissatisfied with parts of her life and her relationship, then balancing her hormones will only help so much. This is the time when she needs a sensitive partner who is willing to make whatever changes are needed to preserve and improve their relationship.

A woman's self-esteem is multi-faceted and how she feels about her sexuality is a huge part of it all. With menopause and all its changes bombarding her, it is no surprise that her libido can drop like a lead balloon. This is not only distressing to the woman, but to her man as well. Low libido resulting in little or no interest in sex (or any aspect of sexuality) doesn't play favorites; it crosses age brackets, lifestyles and all races indiscriminately. A drop in sexual desire signals a fundamental imbalance in a woman's life. To complicate matters, women whose libido has seemingly gone on vacation are not prone to discuss the issue with anyone.

Many factors affect the sex drive. Physical health plays a large role in the overall picture, with hormonal balance being primary—especially levels of estrogen, testosterone, and dopamine. Emotional health allows a woman to experience intimacy deeply. A healthy self-image gives a woman the freedom to fully experience and explore her sexuality. Her sense of her spiritual side adds yet another depth to the experience of sex. If any one of these areas of a woman's life is not functioning well, her sexuality suffers—and so does her sex life. (Those are two different things, by the way.) Her husband also suffers. Having a healthy relationship (including a sexual relationship) means being willing to be vulnerable, and an emotionally challenged perimenopausal or menopausal woman is already feeling *very* vulnerable. What she doesn't need is *more* vulnerability, so she opts out of sex as a protective measure.

For many women enduring a difficult menopause, sex is simply not an option. They don't feel like it, their bodies and psyches aren't craving it, and they aren't thinking of their partners' needs at that point. The need is simply not there, nor is the desire.

For a woman, desire begins in the mind. If a woman is not feeling good about herself (for whatever reason), desire declines or disappears totally. This situation can be the launching pad for an anger attack on the unsuspecting man with whom she has a rela-tionship. Withholding sex is a logical choice for expressing that anger without having to talk about it. It may not be verbally expressed and she may be unin-tentionally punishing him without realizing that is what she's doing. It doesn't matter what she is angry about. (She herself might not even know why she's angry!) A low libido can be a catch-all reason for avoiding relationship issues. Strange and illogical as it is, rejecting her partner gives a woman a measure of control in a situation that defies logic: menopause.

Vaginal dryness, hot flashes, night sweats and interrupted sleep all contribute to a loss of libido and make intercourse painful and uncomfortable. When a woman has low testosterone she is less apt to want sex.

Feelings of frustration, resentment or anger that often accompany menopause can put the damper on a woman's sexual desire. Another factor that contributes to a woman's lack of interest in sex is gravity: After a certain age, everything sags. Hair turns gray or white. Wrinkles appear where they never were before. Shallow wrinkles and fine lines begin to resemble The Grand Canyon.

With all the emphasis on physical beauty and a youthful appearance, women over 40 tend to think their bodies are not as attractive as they were before and they are self-conscious about them. The truth is there is no medical reason why women cannot enjoy an active and fulfilling sex life for their entire lives. A few years ago the CBS show 60 Minutes did a segment on sex over sixty. One man they interviewed said, "It's very simple: What we used to do all night now takes us all night to do." (Obviously keeping a sense of humor helps the situation as well.)

Most men are not interested in just being roommates with their wives. Not only do they need the physical release of sex, they also need the feeling of connectedness it brings—the sense of intimacy. A man who isn't having sex with the woman he loves feels rejected. Sexuality is essential to a man for him to feel emotionally close to his wife. It's also essential to his self-image, so a man who hears night after night, "Not tonight, Honey," gets the idea that his wife is physically punishing him and he cannot understand why she is so uncaring and cold. He believes she is using sex as a weapon. Sometimes that does happen, but most of the time women are not withholding sex in order to get even with their husbands. Sometimes they are hurt because they don't feel loved and appreciated and the feelings of resentment and anger get in the way.

Strange as it may sound, it isn't always the woman who withholds sex. Sometimes it's the man. The partner who wants more sex usually feels shortchanged. The person who has the lesser sexual need can feel criticized and pressured because he or she is not living up to the spouse's expectations. Then the blaming begins. An underlying bad feeling begins to invade the relationship, no matter how understanding a man tries to be. Without physical intimacy it's next to impossible for a man to feel connected emotionally and spiritually. If the situation continues, it can lead to deep unhappiness in either or both partners, infidelity and divorce, unless both of them agree to live together without sex for whatever reason.

So how do couples get past all this and survive the low-libido doldrums? For women the quickest and easiest solution is to stop blaming her partner and take responsibility for improving the relationship, allowing loving feelings to enter her mind. (The body will most likely follow.) Caressing and touching can put a woman in the mood in a short time. She doesn't need to be in the mood to initiate sex. A man can begin paying more attention to his wife's non-sexual needs: making her feel appreciated, complimenting her on little things, thanking her for all she does for him—these are aphrodisiacs to a woman. The soul of true giving is giving your partner what he or she wants and needs, regardless of how you feel about it. Friendship is also a great turn-on for women, so don't discount the idea of doing some things together just as friends without expecting sex.

Understanding the differences between men and women and their sexual needs is crucial for a healthy marriage relationship, and never more so than during a woman's menopause. One person stated the difference between men and women's sexual natures this way: Men are like microwaves; they heat up quickly and get very hot right away. Women are like crock-pots; they take a long time to get hot, but then they stay hot for a long time.

Unfortunately sometimes nothing works. If you are lucky perhaps you can get your wife to see a specialist who deals with natural hormone replacement (most OBGYNs don't have a clue), but that still takes time to find the right balance. If your wife doesn't seem to care (which is often the case), you may have to take things into your own hands. A man needs to be touched and sometimes just a simple massage once a week will do the trick. (Check out a national, low-cost, high-quality massage franchise called, Massage Envy at www.massageenvy.com.) The point is that if your wife isn't willing or capable of meeting your physical needs for closeness and intimacy, you have to do what you have to do. This may sound selfish but if you expect your wife to meet certain needs and she is incapable of doing so, you will build up a lot of resentment which will only complicate the serious relationship problems that you already face. Yes you want to take care of your wife and be supportive, but you can't forget your own needs, too. If you don't take care of yourself, no one else will.

Keys To Understanding

• *This is the time a woman needs a sensitive partner who is willing to make whatever changes are needed to preserve and improve on their relationship.*

• *Most of the time women are not withholding sex in order to get even with their husbands. Sometimes they are hurt because they don't feel loved and appreciated and the feelings of resentment and anger get in the way.*

• *Pay more attention to your wife's non-sexual needs: make her feel appreciated, compliment her on little things ,and thank her for all she does for you.*

• *Give your partner what she wants and needs, regardless of how you feel about it.*

• *Get your wife to see a specialist who deals with natural hormone replacement.*

FOUR:

Understanding Her Midlife Crisis

"Toto, I've got a feeling we're not in Kansas anymore"
Judy Garland
The Wizard of Oz 1939

Popular opinion has attributed the term midlife crisis to men, but the truth is: every year millions of men *and* women reach this crisis stage of their lives. The interesting thing is that this catharsis of the soul can be totally unrelated to menopause in women; the two events simply happen coincidentally about the same time. Sometimes menopause is totally over before a woman enters a midlife crisis. Menopause may not be the only cause of every change a woman experiences during midlife. A woman can choose to let her midlife crisis completely blindside her, turning her world upside down, or she can greet the crisis head-on and welcome the challenge of turning her life around in a new and exciting direction.

Transformation in middle age is a time for examining values and goals that have helped a person arrive at the mid-point of his or her life—somewhere between the ages of 35 and 55. The crisis part refers to the upheaval and pain caused by the psyche-shattering and turbulent transition from the first half of life to the second half. Most people experience this between their late 40s and early 50s.

Midlife crisis is a time when many women no longer feel secure about life as they have known it up until then, yet they cannot look back without regret, nor look forward without trepidation. There is a sense that nothing is right and that can trigger fear and a sense of foreboding. If the woman has unresolved conflicts from the past, a feeling of lost opportunity (and lost youth), and a perception of reduced options available to her, it can throw her into depression. It is a time of self-doubt and questioning both everything that has gone before and everything that is to come. This is the time both women and men realize they are not going to live forever on this earth, their family life has failed to meet their expectations, and they're not enjoying life as they think they should be. They are uncomfortable, and recognize that what they need is *change.*

Typically this period of upheaval lasts between two to twelve years. For a woman, midlife is a time to look how far she has come and to figure out how she wants to spend the last half of her life, turning obstacles into opportunities. (Many women live well into their late 80s and 90s these days.)

Surprisingly research and studies indicate that even more women than men undergo this reinvention of themselves. The most likely reason that more women than men are experiencing this mid-course correction is that women as a whole are different than they were even 20 years ago. Today many women are the bread-winners in their families (often because they are single parents). Also more women have better incomes than they did two decades ago, with many wives out-earning their husbands and higher numbers of women earning over $100,000 (more than three times as many as 10 years ago). This means women have the financial ability, the acquired skills, and the self-esteem and confidence to explore their frustrations and do something about them. Because they are *able* to handle a mid-course correction in their lives, they choose to do exactly that.

One path many midlife women take is to start their own businesses. They did what they had to do to raise their children and now that they're grown and on their own, the women are ready to spread their wings and try something that belongs totally to them: their idea, their management style, their income and, their responsibility. They see that not as a problem, but as a door swinging open to an independent future. A huge part of the allure is the element of control. Also the idea of learning something new, as well as taking care of themselves financially (if they haven't before then). Many ask themselves, "Why not try my own business? The worst that can happen is that my idea doesn't work and I have to get another job."

Not many women go off the deep end during a midlife crisis. A woman's crisis seems to be more about finally getting to do what she *wants* to do, instead of what she *has* to do. Typically men and women don't react in the same way to midlife crisis. Women seem to make bigger changes than men, and have a more positive attitude about the possibilities open to them. Rather than evaluating career or work-related issues as men do, women seem to gain new insights into who they really are (and who they want to become) through soul-searching. Women experience the same midlife crisis, but it's for different reasons. Some seem to feel that the biggest mistake of midlife would be not having a crisis at all because of the good that comes from the experience of self re-evaluation and revision of goals.

What triggers a midlife crisis? Oddly enough it's more likely to be a stressful event rather than menopause or hormonal changes. The death of a parent, going through a divorce, the exodus of children from the home, or even a job change can set off a bout of soul-searching. Recognizing that their biological clocks are winding down can also bring about a crisis. All of their lives women are taught to be introspective and because of that factor, women know they're unhappy sooner than men recognize their own malaise that precedes male midlife crises.

On the negative end of the spectrum of reactions to midlife, a woman can suddenly feel old and vulnerable, questioning why she even exists and re-evaluating everything from commitments to family and friends to mourning the loss of her ability to have more children. On the positive end, midlife crisis can be a genuinely unexpected gift for a woman. It can be wonderfully freeing, opening up new possibilities to enhance the quality of her life and the depth of her relationships with others. It's a time to try the things she's denied herself in the past. In the process of re-inventing herself for the last half of her life, she may just discover who she really is now that she has lived for a while.

The stereotypical male midlife crisis has generally conjured up images of red sports cars and gorgeous younger women to sit in them. Women are more apt to try what they might have earlier considered reckless behavior: bungee jumping, for example, or hiking alone up the highest mountain they can find. Many women simply try things they've always wanted to do but have put off because of family or work obligations. This re-direction or out-of-character behavior could be as simple as taking French cooking lessons, learning to play the piano, or finally writing that novel that's been stewing on the back burner for years.

Interestingly once women have gone through the crisis period, many of them turn to serving others through the therapeutic arts, or through religion, both of those avenues providing opportunities to share what has been learned in the first half of their lives. This can be very rewarding, as well as beneficial to society.

Contradictory to what seems logical, many midlife women who have a burning desire to finally be able to do something for themselves revert to care-giving and nurturing others—especially women who are at the starting line of their midlife sprint to self-discovery. Apparently rolling up one's sleeves and helping other women who are struggling is the shortest path to one's own self-fulfillment. Those who do, not only feel good about themselves but also feel good about the goodwill and blessings they're spreading around.

Some research indicates that it's normal to have more than one midlife crisis, citing the quarter-life crisis, around age 25 when completing education and moving into responsible adulthood and careers, the midlife crisis around the mid-40s, and the three-quarter-life crisis, around age 60 to 65 when retirement becomes the focus. Please note that in order to retire *from* something it is necessary to retire *to* something! Whenever a life-modulating crisis occurs, it presents the opportunity to start over. Women at these crucial transitions in their lives are redefining what it means to age gracefully and are chasing health, wealth, happiness and service to others with amazing passion. In return they are attaining a new level of fulfillment that simply was not achievable for women until now. For these women, midlife can present their greatest opportunity for personal growth, power, satisfaction and happiness, making the years after midlife the best half of a woman's life. The glass of life is, after all, not half-empty, but half-full.

Keys To Understanding

• *Both men and women can experience a midlife crisis, but for a woman it may or may not be related to menopausal symptoms, although it often is.*

• *Midlife is a time for change, and that can be a good thing. A positive attitude makes all the difference in how a person copes with the switch from what has been to what is to come. Focus on the possibilities.*

• *For many women, midlife is a chance to finally do what she wants to do instead of what it was necessary for her to do for so many years.*

• *Examination of one's self and revision of goals are not negative aspects, but positive features of the midlife years.*

FIVE:

Empty Nest Syndrome

"Houston, we have a problem."
Tom Hanks
Apollo 13 1995

Okay. That's the last one off to college. Now what?

Sometimes the empty-nest syndrome—usually when the last child leaves home for college or gets married—gives a woman the excuse she needs to become her own person, try something new, or reinvent herself. Suddenly the person who has depended on her, confided in her, and shared his or her entire life with mom no longer needs her. Gone are the car pools, shuffling several teenagers back and forth to this practice and that party. The house is suddenly easier to clean, the grocery bill is less, and the laundry hamper is no longer as full as it has been for the last 18 years.

It's interesting that, although parents prepare their children for leaving home by guiding them through college applications and SAT tests, seldom do parents plan ahead to prepare themselves for the day when the child's bedroom is empty and the nest is empty. The best time for the parent to prepare for the day they have the house to themselves is at the same time they are preparing their children to launch out on their own. Working on the marital relationship and making plans of their own for the time when the last child has left is important and builds anticipation and even excitement for the changes to come. Instead of a time of grief and loss, these parents experience a time of renewal and freedom that often revitalizes their relationship. Their attitude is that they are entering the final stage of child-rearing. The truth is that a woman suffering through the empty nest syndrome really hasn't lost anything. Actually she has gained—an adult child who can now begin to truly relate to the struggles and challenges of being an adult that parents experience.

Many women feel a profound sense of loss when the last child leaves home. Sadness, depression, grief, a sense of loss of identity, and even guilt can be natural reactions to the cutting of the cord. Some women find themselves weeping for no apparent reason, or sitting by themselves in the child's former bedroom in order to feel closer. These are natural reactions to this change in a woman's life. The feelings that wash over a woman during this time are nothing to be ashamed of and most women are able to adjust in a short time.

Some, however, do not regroup as quickly. Women experiencing severe symptoms (lasting longer than a week or two) could be feeling that their useful lives are over, or they are so sad and depressed that they don't want to mix with friends or even go to work. Crying could be excessive for these women.

To complicate the situation, many women whose last child has fled the nest may also be experiencing menopause. Self-confidence may be out the window. And it is not unusual for these same women to be also dealing with increasingly dependent elderly parents— a triple whammy, for sure. It's a time of life when a woman is especially vulnerable.

So what's a woman left in this empty nest to do?

Counseling could certainly help, as could natural supplements and bioidentical or natural hormones. Maintaining communication with the child (or children) is very important, but it's also important to not overdo it. The child is trying to take his or her first major move into adulthood, and it can be scary, but it's also necessary. Keeping a journal can be helpful for women during this time. When a distraught and lonely mother writes out her feelings and concerns on paper, she can help give the child room to try his or her wings without hovering too protectively. E-mail can also be a good way to communicate as long as it doesn't require the child to respond in the mother's timeframe and the messages are kept brief. It's all about freedom for the child and restraint and restructuring for the mother. It's time for the mother to begin thinking about who she is (or would like to be) now that she has all this freedom to enter a new phase of her life. This is the time to develop a relationship with the adult child. This is a time for new and exciting beginnings, not a time for endings—for both the child and the mother, who are both discovering new independence. Every woman in this situation has a choice to make: moan and groan about the perceived losses, or move ahead and grow as a person.

This is also a perfect time for a woman to rediscover her husband—when they are free to concentrate on each other. All of those things they talked about doing *someday* can now be explored. Lucky the couple that planned ahead for this day! The key to not just surviving the empty nest years but actually thriving in them as a couple is to build and strengthen your relationship *before* the nest empties.

Preparation for the empty nest phase of a relationship with one's spouse involves a commitment to let go of the past and work together to make the coming years the best ones of all. With the children out of the house couples will now have time to focus on each other and their values and goals. Communication is especially important when it's just one woman and one man in the house. This is the time for forgiveness of the past, honesty with each other, and commitment to giving the years ahead the best effort possible from each partner. It's also the time for the friendship between a man and wife to flourish and deepen. The absence of the children in the house makes that more possible than it has been before.

These years can be the best and most rewarding in an entire marriage. It's as if life is saying, "Go ahead. Enjoy each other and have fun together. You've done it all. Now relax together and get closer than ever. Pass along what you've learned to help other couples who might be struggling. Give something back. Strengthen your physical relationship and your spiritual connection." Looking at this time as simply another adjustment in a life-long relationship helps put the empty nest in perspective.

Keys To Understanding

• *Planning ahead for the day when the nest is empty builds anticipation and excitement for the changes to come.*

• *Sometimes three elements come together to create the perfect storm: menopause, the emptying of the nest and a midlife crisis.*

• *Let go of the past and work with your wife to make the years ahead the best you've ever shared.*

• *Rediscover each other and learn to appreciate who you are now by building on the years you've already spent together.*

• *Share what you've learned over your married years with other couples who may be experiencing turmoil in their relationships.*

PART TWO
COPING

SIX:

What Women Should Do

"Snap out of it."
Cher
Moonstruck 1987

Even if your wife doesn't seem interested in reading anything you suggest, it would be a good idea for you to have some thoughts on how to help her through menopause or other midlife issues. (If she would read just this one chapter in this book, it should improve things for both of you.)

The good news is women do *not* need to just sit there without being proactive. There's nothing like knowledge to dispel fear and worry. Understanding what is happening to a woman's body and mind during this time is the key to coping with the changes that occur. So the first thing women can do to help themselves is to be aware of what is happening and why.

Many doctors prescribe synthetic hormones and prescription antidepressants, but women should explore readily available natural antidepressants and supplements to help them through this difficult time in their lives.

Having hormone levels checked is another major step in *managing* menopause (as opposed to just *surviving* it by reacting to the changes as they happen). A woman's hormone levels can begin shifting in the 30s and 40s and shift dramatically during the late 40s and 50s. That's why it's very important for women to start testing their hormone levels in their mid- to late 30s.

There are three basic ways of testing hormone levels: through the blood, urine or saliva. Tests using these methods are readily available. Saliva testing is very reliable for measuring hormone levels. It costs less than blood tests, can be done at home by collecting saliva four times in one day, and involves no needles or stress. Hormone levels in saliva remain stable for several days, and the results of the tests can be mailed back to your health care provider or to you if you purchase a test from an independent lab. The major hormones tested in either blood or saliva are estrogen, progesterone, testosterone, DHEA, cortisol, and Human Growth Hormone or IGF-1.

Urine tests are also very accurate. Urine testing allows direct measurement of free (or available) hormone levels, but it also measures hormone metabolites which indicate the effects of hormones on the body. Consequently urine testing provides much more information than any other hormone testing process. Some doctors will also want a complete serum test to get a complete reading on everything happening in a woman's body, but for hormone testing, urine is very good, very accurate and can be done in the comfort of one's home.

It's impossible to overestimate the importance of healthy hormone balance. Hormones are chemicals produced within the body and released into the bloodstream by the endocrine glands. Their purpose is to regulate body functions—everything from sleep patterns to bone structure, mood swings, fatigue, dizziness, decreased memory, weight control, acne, normal sex drive, thinning hair or hair where you don't want it, menstrual cycles and reproduction. Unbalanced hormones can make feeling good impossible and make a woman look older than she is by affecting the condition of her skin, hair, bones, and energy level. Estrogen is the primary female hormone; progesterone and testosterone are also vitally important to a woman's wellbeing, testosterone being the hormone that can promote and sustain a satisfying sex life throughout a lifetime. Testosterone is also vitally important for a woman's bones and heart. There are more testosterone receptors in the heart than in any other part of the body. An optimal testosterone level is important to a woman on many levels other than libido.

Hormone Replacement Therapy is a phrase every woman over thirty has heard, and many have tried it. Since hormone replacement affects every single cell in the body, it's pretty important to get it right. Years ago those original replacement hormones were synthesized from the urine of pregnant horses (and still are), which *were* natural—but only to other horses. Studies have proven that many women who used this type of hormone replacement now suffer from more heart disease, osteoporosis, senility and other debilitations. One product carries a printed warning of a possible link to endometrial carcinoma.

The obvious answer is to use *bioidentical* hormone replacements. (See Chapter Eight.) As this book is being written the FDA is instructing compounding pharmacies that they can no longer use the term bioidentical. In fact they are also telling compounding pharmacies that they can no longer use a natural hormone (estriol) in formulating prescriptions. Since estriol is a key component in many prescriptions, this could jeopardize the care that many women have been receiving. The fact is that a major drug company (Wyeth), has pressured the FDA for years to control compounding pharmacies. As more women have moved toward natural hormone replacement, the big drug companies have lost sales. This is going to be a major battle as women and their doctors fight to keep natural hormone therapy a viable option for hormonally challenged women.

Bioidentical hormones are made from hormone precursors found in yams and soybeans. Their molecular structure is a duplication of the human hormones they are replacing. They are truly bioidentical—exactly the same as those in women's bodies. Since they have all the benefits offered by the synthetic hormones, it simply makes sense to use bioidentical hormones for replacement therapy.

The advantages of taking bioidentical replacement hormones are many, including:

- Prevention of osteoporosis.
- Restoration of bone strength.
- Fewer hot flashes.
- Less vaginal dryness and/or thinning.
- Protection against stroke and heart disease.
- Improved cholesterol levels.
- Better sleep (putting them in a better mood).
- Improved memory and concentration.
- Improved sex drive (libido).
- Less risk of depression, endometrial and breast cancer.

Beyond estrogens and progesterone are other hormones such as DHEA and testosterone. (Yes, women have that, too! And men have some estrogen and progesterone, usually thought of as female hormones. In fact, the average 55 year old male has more estrogen than the average 55 year old female.) The FDA is also now restricting the importation of DHEA into this country. Here is another vital natural hormonal supplement that may be forced off the shelves.

But hormone replacement is only part of the solution to the problems associated with menopause. It's also vitally important that thyroid levels be optimal. Thyroid is the most misunderstood hormone. If your thyroid levels aren't right, you could have a host of problems. In many instances a patient's primary care physician will notice low normal thyroid levels through blood, urine or saliva tests and not suggest any action because the physican considers the levels normal. Low normal levels are not optimal levels, and sometimes simple treatment with thyroid hormone replacement will lead to significant symptom improvement. Women in general experience more thyroid issues than men. Another common deficiency found in women and men is low levels of iodine. Iodine helps regulate thyroid levels. Low thyroid levels can even influence self-esteem and self-worth so it is something that shouldn't be overlooked as optimal throid levels are vitally important.

Eating healthy foods is another way to improve health and increase resilience. A diet rich in fresh, whole foods (rather than packaged and canned foods) is a step in the right direction. Eliminating food colors, synthetics flavorings, chemicals and preservatives will increase the body's ability to adapt and better cope with the stresses of menopause. (It wouldn't hurt the entire family's health, either!) Replacing artificial sweeteners with fresh fruits and vegetables also helps.

Because of the many changes their bodies and psyches are going through during menopause, some women want absolutely nothing to do with the physical part of marriage. Hot flashes, night sweats, and other physical changes in their own bodies are embarrassing to them and keep them from enjoying intimacy to the extent they did previously. (Those are the last things on men's minds when they're in a sexual frame of mind and are far less important to men than they are to women.) Granted it's an important part of marriage, but recognizing that the physical part is only a *part* of it and not the *whole* of it is important. When women are temporarily not interested in sexual intimacy, they could explore the friendship aspect of their relationships with their husbands. Not all women opt out of sex during menopause, however.

Cutting husbands out of their lives is not the answer, either. Talking to her husband is something proactive a woman can do to help herself through this time. Sharing what she is experiencing—her worries and her fears as well—often deepens the marriage relationship. At the very least, it makes the husband feel less left out in the cold. At the very best, it will keep the communication lines open and enable him to feel that he is helping her through this transition time in some way.

Because menopause is not just physical but also emotional, it is equally important that a woman find a therapist who offers short-term solutions and concentrates on the present and the future instead of revisiting all the bad times and events and trying to resolve the past.   The past is exactly that: PAST. Concentrating on the goal instead of the past is a healthier exercise.

The truth is that a menopausal woman feels everything more keenly during this time in her life. It's as if her senses are heightened and her emotions are very close to the surface. She is often weepy and doesn't have a good explanation of why. Or something that apparently didn't irritate her for years now drives her wild and she explodes for apparently no reason. The truth is she's been irritated before, but has suppressed her feelings. It's not uncommon for old wounds to open and old battles to be fought once again because she cannot hold her feelings in as well as she did before menopause. Anger surfaces and bursts out at the most inopportune moments.

Anxiety is common, especially just before the beginning of a hot flash. Men need to refrain from discounting any feeling a woman expresses during the transition years of perimenopause and menopause. A feeling is a feeling and saying it's unimportant or ridiculous won't make it go away. It will only make a wife feel that her husband truly doesn't understand her. This would be a good time for a woman to tell (warn) her husband how she's feeling so he can feel like part of the solution, not part of the problem.

The companion to anxiety is depression, causing a woman to think in self-destructive patterns, which causes deeper depression. Irregularities in estrogen affect neurotransmitters, the mood-regulators of the body. (See the next chapter.) If a woman is feeling anxious or depressed, the medical community is often quick to treat the symptom and ignore the cause. Pharmaceutical anti-depressants are often readily prescribed to fix the surface problem and all too often nothing is done about the underlying cause: hormonal inbalance.

Between the ages of 35 and 55 it's very important that women have health providers who will work with them—a *partner* approach to solving health issues. A good idea is to set up a separate appointment to discuss only issues and ask questions about menopause. Ask for at least 15 minutes for this appointment and spend some time preparing your questions before you arrive for the appointment. Any woman is the best source of knowledge about her own body, including what works for her and what doesn't. She needs to trust herself and her intuition and utilize the health practitioner's specialized expertise to get specific information and answers. Some doctors encourage women to prepare and maintain a menopause diary.

At this appointment a woman should be prepared to discuss her periods in detail: when they started, what they were like when she was a teenager, how long the periods last, and if there is spotting between periods. A history of contraception and pregnancies and past medical history is important, too, including surgeries and chronic illnesses. Ditto for family history. A list of the medications and any supplements the woman is taking, as well as the amounts of caffeine and alcohol she consumes and how much she smokes are also important pieces of information. Amounts and frequency of exercise and sexual history are also helpful indicators for the menopause diary as well. A woman who knows her own strengths and weaknesses and her desires will help the health care provider put together a plan for coping with menopause with as little disruption as possible. It will be a valuable 15 minutes for everyone—including the anxious and caring husband of the menopausal woman.

The biggest key is to find someone who understands and practices hormone balancing. Many doctors have entered this field, but there are very few real experts who know what they are doing in this area of medicine. It is vitally important for a woman to find someone who is qualified and experienced in hormone replacement who can help her through this challenging period.

Keys To Understanding

• *The first thing women can do to help themselves through menopause is to be aware of what is happening and why.*

• *Find a doctor who understands and prescribes bioidentical hormone replacement therapy.*

• *Eat healthy foods to improve health and increase resilience.*

• *If a woman can share what she is experiencing (including her worries and fears), the marriage relationship can often be deepened. At the very least it makes the husband feel less left out in the cold.*

• *Keep the communication lines open to make the husband feel he is helping her in some way.*

SEVEN:

Maybe It's The Neurotransmitters

"Well, nobody's perfect."
Joe E. Brown
Some Like it Hot 1959

According to figures from the National Institute of Mental Health one out of every 10 American adults suffers from some form of depression each year. That translates into almost 40 million Americans. Depression hits both men and women, but about twice as many women seem to be more affected by it. In 2007, revenues from prescriptions for antidepressants soared to over $20 billion worldwide. Over 12 million prescriptions were written for children between the ages of 0-17, with the fastest growing segment being children ages five and younger.

Depression symptoms include a sense of worthlessness, feeling suicidal, feelings of hopelessness, fluctuating weight, either not being able to sleep or sleeping all the time, inability to concentrate, short-term memory problems, restlessness and sadness. Prescriptions for depression of all types are normally treated with counseling and/or antidepressants, depending on the severity of the case. Usually the medication has to be taken from nine months to two-and-a-half years. Some people remain on them for life.

Some of the usually prescribed medications produce side-effects such as anxiety (the very thing they are supposed to alleviate!), dryness of the mouth, headaches, loss of sexual desire and weight variances both upward and downward.

Everyone has feelings of sadness or disappointment from time to time. But when the feelings are extreme (such as apathy or despair), and won't go away, the root cause may be depression, resulting in an inability to work or enjoy life, or even to eat or sleep properly.

Depression is not age-specific; it affects people of all ages and is expressed in different ways, depending on the age, sex and culture of the person experiencing it. An elderly man in a nursing home does not usually have the same symptoms of depression as a young woman who is hostile and out of sorts with everyone. Twice as many women experience depression as men do, with symptoms of guilt feelings, overeating, and wanting to just crawl into bed and sleep all the time.

A large portion of depression and anxiety disorders can be attributed to a chemical imbalance called

Neurotransmitter Deficiency Disorder, or NDD. Symptoms of NDD can include anorexia, attention deficit disorder, anxiety, bulimia, chronic fatigue, depression, fibromyalgia, insomnia, irritable bowel syndrome, learning disorders, menopausal symptoms, migraines, obesity, panic attacks and PMS.

Neurotransmitters are specialized, naturally occurring chemical substances in the brain. Simply put, they transfer messages from the neurons (nerve cells) in the form of electrical impulses which transform to chemical impulses and back to electrical impulses from one cell to another to control specialized activities. The human brain has between 10 billion to 100 billion neurons. All of these impulses move amazingly fast, allowing the brain to respond in an instant.

About 30 neurotransmitters have been identified. Serotonin, norepinephrine, dopamine, epinephrine, Histamine, acetylcholine and GABA are the most common ones. Serotonin, norepinephrine and dopamine operate in the areas of the brain that govern emotions, reactions to stress, sleep, appetite and sexuality. Neurotransmitters can be out of balance, affecting mood, sleep, weight, digestion, and behavior.

Common antidepressant drugs such as Prozac, Zoloft and Paxil offer *temporary* solutions to the symptoms of depression by rearranging the body's neurotransmitters. This class of drugs is called SSRI (selective serotonin re-uptake inhibitors). They don't add any neurotransmitters. Once the drug is discontinued, the problem of unbalanced neurotransmitters returns.

Several factors contribute to low levels of neurotransmitters, including poor diet—and consequently poor nutrition—stress overload, and environmental influences. A person with NDD (neurotransmitter deficiency disorder) can exhibit these indicators: anxiety, chronic fatigue, fibromyalgia, insomnia, learning difficulties, panic attacks, migraine headaches, premenstrual syndrome and menopausal problems.

A balanced diet with enough fats, carbohydrates and protein is essential to maintaining neurotransmitter health. Alcohol, nicotine and excess caffeine are neurotoxins and should be avoided. Since most neurotransmitters are made from protein, it's critical to consume enough protein in the diet (between 40 to 70 grams daily for non-athletes). Carbohydrates help with tryptophan absorption which helps raise serotonin levels. Diets high in protein and low in carbohydrates decrease levels of serotonin. This is especially important to women, since they tend to have one-third less serotonin than men. High protein foods such as fish, chicken, dairy products, almonds, avocados, bananas, legumes, soy products, pumpkin and sesame seeds promote the production of the neurotransmitter dopamine.

There are reports of good success at raising neurotransmitter levels through alternative methods such as herbs, yoga, massage, hypnosis, acupuncture, meditation and reflexology. One type of treatment that has produced excellent results is amino acid neurotransmitter therapy (AANT). Taking amino acid precursors to the neurotransmitters in the form of supplements has resulted in naturally increased levels of neurotransmitters as the body replenishes them to proper levels. Through amino acid neurotransmitter therapy 5HTP is converted into serotonin and eventually into melatonin. Phenylalanine becomes tyrosine and eventually dopamine as well as L-Dopa, norepinephrine and epinephrine. Which amino acids are recommended depends upon the person's individual needs based upon the levels of neurotransmitters uncovered by a simple urine test to measure levels of epinephrine, norepinephrine, dopamine, serotonin, GABA, PEA, histamine and others.

A person who has been taking SSRI drugs can begin amino acid therapy while being gradually and safely weaned off the SSRI medications. There are no known side effects of amino acid neurotransmitter therapy other than minor nausea, cramping or diarrhea in less than 5% of the people on AANT, and those people had severe neurotransmitter deficiency. If those symptoms should occur, the amino acids are stopped, and once symptoms disappear, a very low dosing is begun and gradually increased over a period of several weeks. That process is normally very effective.

Every individual responds differently to the same treatment, of course, but most people on AANT notice marked improvement in their moods within a few days. Some people need several months to notice gradual improvements.

Amino acid neurotransmitter therapy can make an incredible difference in a person's emotional outlook and overall health. If the body doesn't have what it needs to do the various jobs it's required to do, the person isn't going to feel well. It's that simple.

Keys To Understanding

• Twice as many women experience depression as men do, with symptoms of guilt feelings, overeating, and wanting to just crawl into bed and sleep all the time.

•Neurotransmitters can be out of balance affecting mood, behavior, sleep, weight, digestion, emotions, reactions to stress, and sexuality.

• Common antidepressant drugs such as Prozac, Zoloft and Paxil offer temporary solutions to the symptoms of depression but they don't add any neuro-transmitters and once the drug is stopped, the imbalance returns.

• Symptoms of NDD (Neurotransmitter Deficiency Disorder) are anxiety, chronic fatigue, fibromyalgia, insomnia, learning difficulties, panic attacks, migraine headaches, premenstrual syndrome and menopausal problems, to name a few.

• There is a test to determine if a person has NDD. Any peri-menopausal or menopausal woman would be wise to take it.

Note: This *chapter is based on a booklet entitled Neurotransmitter Deficiency Disorder by Bill Anton, published by Age Diagnostic Laboratories. (See Bibliography at the end of this book.)*

EIGHT:

What Men Can Do—The Power of One

"You make me want to be a better man."
Jack Nicholson
As Good As it Gets 1997

Many women dealing with the emotional and physical upheavals in their lives during this time do not have the patience or desire to go to a counselor or therapist. You can go alone. There is much you can do by yourself to turn your situation around, support your wife, and end up happy—and still married. Divorce is not the answer. No matter how stressed out you both are, no matter how bad things are right now, you can survive this and still be together.

Here are some strategies you can begin using right now that will both ease the tension between you and your wife and begin to turn the situation around for you. The good news is that you do not have to just sit by and watch all this happening to your wife and to your relationship. If your wife is enduring menopause and your relationship is suffering, you do not have to go belly-up and just let it fall apart. You've invested far too much time, effort and emotion into your marriage, and there are many strategies you can implement to save it. You can start right now and you can do it on your own. Don't try to do them all at once. Just pick one or two and try to integrate them into your life. Then try one or two other techniques. Not everything will work for everyone, so don't give up too soon. If one strategy doesn't work in your situation, try another one.

Don't take it personally. While she is experiencing menopausal symptoms, a woman's feelings and symptoms run the gamut. And they can change so quickly it makes both her head and yours spin. Mood swings, physical exhaustion and feelings of insecurity, anxiousness and overwhelming sadness are not unusual. In a sense she's grieving the loss of her youth and her sense of identity. If the children are at the point of leaving home, add in the empty-nest syndrome. Encouraging her to talk with you about all of this may be more than she can handle because she probably hasn't solidified how she feels about it. Just be there for her when she is ready to talk.

Put thoughts of divorce out of your mind. You may think you're at the end of your rope, but you are not there yet. Giving up and getting out is not the answer. Divorce has repercussions that last. (For example if you have children together, you will always have that parental connection with your spouse. That doesn't go away.) Divorce also doesn't free you from the emotional grip of your ex-spouse. Giving up without trying to work through the problem means the unresolved issue is carried into the next relationship with you. You owe it to yourself, your wife, and your children to try alternatives to solving your relationship problems first. Divorce doesn't go away. Most marriages can be changed, and are worth changing. But be prepared: It will require hard work!

Remember that it's not *your* body that's changing daily. Most women don't want their husbands to take charge and try to fix things when it comes to menopause. You can suggest and point her in the right direction for helpful books and other resources, but this is happening to her, not you. There is no possible way you can truly understand what she is living with right now, so accept that and be as supportive as you can.

Consider focusing on possible solutions rather than on why you have a problem. There is a type of therapy that does exactly that and it has helped save thousands of seemingly hopeless marriages. It's called Solution-Oriented Brief Therapy. A therapist who specializes in this method usually doesn't see clients for more than four to six sessions. You enter into it, knowing there is an end in sight. Time is not spent on delving into the past nor on *he did/she did* conversations to find out why things are in the present state in the relationship. Everyone's efforts are focused on the desired result: a repaired relationship. If your wife will not attend, you can still go through the therapy alone and achieve amazing results in your relationship. Never underestimate the power of one!

Concentrate on what you do that she accepts and appreciates and stop doing things that she rejects (even if she used to like those things). If your wife reacts badly to your continued suggestions that you go to bed and work on your relationship, stop suggesting it. If she pushes you away when you try to hug her, don't try to hug her. Remember this is what's happening right now; it probably won't last forever. When you make small adjustments, the dynamics of the relationship change and that can produce the results you want. Small changes can work big results. And you *can* get through it!

Criticism and complaining are ineffective. They won't get your relationship with your wife back where it was before menopause broad-sided you.

Don't say, *My wife is going through menopause.* Instead shift your attitude to *We're going through menopause.* This one strategy alone will not only help her, but you as well. It means you're in this battle together. Neither of you will feel that it's just you against the world. It's the *two* of you against the world.

Find something positive you can do for your wife that you know would please her (not something *you* think she needs). For example, if she likes a type of music you can't stand, buy her a CD of the kind she likes. (And maybe buy yourself some earplugs.)

Don't nag or push. Asking your wife to do something she is now uncomfortable doing (even if she used to do it before), will push her away and won't accomplish what you really want.

Ignore her negative comments. If they are something you feel you cannot ignore, wait until the moment has passed before you mention the incident, if you mention it at all. Marriage is long-term and long-term is made up of accumulated moments. Ask yourself if you can live with the negative comments while your wife is going through this emotional upheaval.

Speak softly when you bring up a problem area in your relationship. This will help keep the situation from escalating. Women tend to equate intimacy with communication skills.

Don't react to something she says or does in a passive-aggressive manner. It will only undo all the good you've been trying to do. Your wife may be expecting you to react a certain way. Change your response and surprise her by being open to what she's saying.

If she misinterprets something you said, don't argue with her. A quick way to diffuse a budding argument is to be the generous one and say you're not sure exactly what you said, and then say something like, "This is what I *meant* to say."

Avoid arguments about money. Your wife will interpret it as your trying to control her. *Remember that all couples have problems.* Her menopause just blows them out of proportion.

Be sensual instead of sexual. Backrubs, walks on the beach, sitting together on the couch in front of a fire—all of these work toward relieving a woman's anxiety about having sex during a time when she doesn't feel like it.

This would be a good time to put your relationship ahead of your individual desires. This will relieve some of the pressure you are both feeling.

Show her that you honor and respect her by recognizing all the little things she does to make life better for you. Recognition and acceptance pave the way to peace.

Don't confuse what you need with what you want. They aren't the same thing.

Your relationship is the most important thing. (Forget about proving who forgot to put the dog out because she is having trouble concentrating these days.)

Don't defend yourself. Learn to duck any criticisms your wife may hurl at you when she's upset. You can diffuse a potential bomb by saying something such as, "You could be right."

Take care of yourself as much as you can. If she forgets to iron your shirt, either do it yourself or ask her to show you how to do it. Do something totally out of character. It will surprise both of you!

Give your wife all the space she needs, as often as she needs it. Even if you don't like it.

Take one step back. Realize that you cannot fix all your wife's problems during menopause. Accept that and do what you can to make this transition time as easy as possible for her. She's not in control; her body is. Trying to be Mr. Fix-It is not the path to take right now. Hopefully her body will straighten itself out eventually with proper medical care. You just need to be supportive while that's happening.

Try to keep your perspective. The current situation won't last forever. Putting your wife's needs first exhibits true love—even if her need is space to be by herself instead of with you.

Change your thinking (and speech) to plural instead of singular. Your wife may be experiencing menopause, but you are going through it, too, right alongside her. Saying "We're going through menopause." means you are right there for her, helping her cope with the changes she's experiencing.

Look for things you can do to express your caring and concern for your wife without thought of reward or acknowledgement. You *do* have the inner strength to bring about change in your relationship. (We're not talking about bringing home a dozen roses for her. We're talking about taking the garbage out without being asked—or something else she usually has to ask you to do.) If she doesn't notice, you'll have the satisfaction of knowing you did something positive to begin the process of a mid-course correction in your relationship.

Stop an argument in its tracks by simply saying, "I understand." (Even if you don't completely understand, you know she's upset and needs to vent.)

Read books on the subject of menopause so you'll understand how menopause affects women. It will help you as well. Also bear in mind that just as every woman is different, so is every menopause. Your wife is an individual and she may or may not respond to typical menopausal reactions as the books say she will. Some women hardly experience any difficulties at all; others seem to have every symptom known to womankind. Avoiding the problem doesn't work. Knowing why your wife is behaving in a totally different way than you've ever seen will help you help her through it as well as let you know that you are not to blame for the situation. (See the Bibliography at the end of the book for a recommended reading list.)

The single-most important thing your wife needs from you is your understanding. She cannot control the changes in her body without help. She needs to know that you understand that and that you are not blaming her for the difference it is making in your relationship. She will appreciate that more than she can express to you, so don't set a time limit on your understanding.

Menopause is not just an ending; it's also a beginning. Once she's on the other side of this huge change, she just might surprise you with her new freedom and attitudes and you'll fall in love with her all over again.

Resistance doesn't work. Yes things are changing. Yes you aren't thrilled with the situation. But expressing your desire for things to go back the way they were before menopause will work against you. If you can ride the roller coaster for the duration, you stand a better chance of saving your marriage.

Affirm your wife's inner worth. She is most likely feeling like a reject and a failure during the menopausal changes happening to her. It's a time of revaluation and trying to figure out who she is now.

Try to not take the situation personally. It's not about sex or love. It's about her biology.

Put on a happy face. If you act angry about the changes in your marriage due to her menopause, what would make her want to be with you? If you act happy, you are more apt to feel better and she will pick up on that.

Try to keep your sense of humor. Remember that you are not getting any younger, either.

Give up your right to be right. Keep your eye on the goal: a restored relationship.

Accept her need to be alone. She needs time to process all the changes she's experiencing—not only physically, but emotionally, too.

Tell your wife that you are on her side, no matter what. You're in this together.

Pick your battles, and pick the timing of them. No doubt there will be issues that arise that you will need to discuss, whether they are unpleasant or not. Try to be aware of her moods and keep anger or hurt feelings out of the discussion.

Remind yourself that the relationship is more important than getting what you want right now. Your goal is to save the relationship and get it back on firm footing.

Find other ways to feel connected to your wife other than sex. Because a woman's hormones are in chaos, sex may be the last thing she wants. If that's the case, try sharing intimate memories you experienced together. Intimacy doesn't necessarily mean sex; it can be just a recollection of a wonderful time of feeling really connected as you walked on the beach, or experienced a special event or moment together. Remembering the times you've shared that special connection between you will help you over the rough moments.

Compliment your wife frequently. Substitute a compliment when you feel a complaint ready to pop out of your mouth.

Accept your wife as she is now. Don't keep pointing out how she used to be. It's counterproductive. She will see it as a criticism and as your wanting your way.

Be forgiving. Forgive her, and forgive yourself. Resentment and bitterness are killers. No one ever died from being too forgiving.

Create harmony every chance you get. Just enjoying a movie in the same room can be peaceful and harmonious.

Remember why you're making these changes in yourself and your behavior. It's not in order for you to get your own needs met. It's so that you can support your wife in a difficult time. If you can do that selflessly, your reward should be great.

Work on your own areas that need improving. While your wife is dealing with raging hormones and hot flashes (or whatever symptoms she's experiencing), pinpoint a few things you can do to make yourself a better husband. Menopause can last anywhere from a few months to a few years, so these should be permanent changes you know you should make in yourself anyway, not just something you try for a few months until your wife gets over her menopause. She'll notice the changes but even if she doesn't say anything to you, you'll know you're a better person for having made the effort. That in itself will make a change in how you relate to your wife.

Remind yourself that your wife is not choosing to do this on purpose. Stop blaming her and stop making yourself the victim.

Adopt a commonsense approach and learn as much as you can about what is happening to your wife. Knowledge is the key to change.

Accept menopause as a chance to strengthen your relationship by understanding, being patient, and expressing love in small non-sexual ways.

The greatest need your wife has right now is your understanding. Simply saying, "I understand. How can I help?" will lighten the tension.

Tell her you love her in both verbal and non-verbal ways. She's probably not feeling very loveable right now.

Encourage her to tell you what's bothering her. Don't make light of it or shrug it off as if it's foolish for her to get hung up on whatever it is. Acknowledge her feelings and assure her that you'll get through this together.

Tell her how much you value the wisdom that age brings with it. Let her know she's much more valuable to you now that you've been through so much together over the years.

Accept your own aging. Prove it by throwing out your hair-coloring supplies. No woman wants to look older than her husband! There's something really beautiful about growing old together.

Do NOT tell her you don't mind the little pot belly she's developed! And don't remind her she needs to exercise and eat right to stay slim. (If she gains a few pounds, she can also lose it later.)

Listen to her. Hear her out when she talks about something you're not interested in hearing. Be thoughtful how you respond to something she's said. Respond in a non-critical way. For example, she says, "I feel so old! Like my life is almost over! The kids are gone and I don't know who I am anymore." Your incorrect response would be, "That's foolish! You'll never be old." Your correct response would be, "I understand. Sometimes I feel the same way, but I know we have wonderful years ahead of us. And I certainly know who you are; you're the woman I love with all my heart." (Or something similar. Use your imagination!)

If she has expressed a sense of loss at not being able to have more children, remind her that she will always be a mother. That will never change.

Back off and let her menopause run its course. She can't stop it and neither can you, so you might as well roll with it.

View menopause not as an ending, but as a transition to another stage of life.

Discuss with her the advice she's getting from her doctors. The more you know, the more you can help her. And she might be relieved to be able to talk to you about it all.

Support her without being judgmental. She may not want to hear your opinion, so just listen to her. (That means giving her your undivided attention.) If she asks for your opinion, use a friendly tone, not a dictatorial one. It's her body and, ultimately, her decision on how she cares for it.

Ask her how she would like you to support her, both physically and emotionally. Find out how you can support her and do it her way, not yours.

Let her know you accept her decision (even if you disagree with it) and be there for her.

Don't buy her a lot of books to read about menopause and related subjects. She's already overwhelmed and that will only make her feel that you're trying to force your opinion on her. You can suggest a good book you heard about that you thought might help her, but sharing information is different from pressuring her to read what pushes your viewpoint.

Let her make her own decisions. When you try to take charge and fix things for her, it only drives a wedge between you. You can't *fix* menopause. She has to go through it. But you can make things easier for her by following these suggestions: Listen, talk, ask how you can help. Don't act as if something's broken. She'll see it as condescending. She's not broken; she's just making huge adjustments and she *will* get *through* it.

Give her time alone to process everything that's happening to her. She'll need more alone time than she's been used to in order to take care of her own inner needs.

Do your share of the household responsibilities without being asked and do them with a cheerful attitude. Do them because you want to help.

Put your wife's needs ahead of your own, but not in order to get your own needs met. Take care of your own needs as well.

Don't make all these changes at once. (You don't want to give your wife a heart-attack!)

Keys To Understanding

• *Don't say, My wife is going through menopause. Instead say, We're going through menopause.*

• *Don't confuse what you need with what you want.*

• *Trying to be Mr. Fix-It is not the path to take right now.*

• *Whatever you do, don't give up!*

• *Remember, this is for now. It's not forever.*

NINE:

Three Types of Therapy That Work

"My mama always said, "Life is like a box of choco-lates; you never know what you're gonna get."
Tom Hanks
Forest Gump 1994

When you're in the middle of a heated argument with a hormonally challenged woman, you may feel that you cannot win. But that is not true. You *can* win. The thing to do is not give in to your anger and frustration at the immediate situation and remember how much you love this woman and how much you want the marriage to succeed.

Consider asking your wife to attend therapy with you. (Don't tell her *she* needs therapy. You *both* need it. You can't be married by yourself!)

There are three types of therapy that do a great job of getting people to move forward instead of back-ward: Solution-Oriented Brief Therapy (SBT), Cognitive Behavior Therapy (CBT) and Imago Relationship Therapy (IRT). All three of these modal-ities are forward-oriented and do not dwell on the past or how you got into the situation you are in. Couples dealing with a disruptive menopause do not have time to explore everything that happened in the past. Time is of the essence to help you cope with the future of your relationship. One of these three types of therapy should be helpful to you. A summary of each follows.

<u>Solution-Oriented Brief Therapy:</u> Solution-Oriented Brief Therapy (SBT) focuses on solutions instead of trying to find out what caused the problem. SBT isn't concerned with why things went wrong, but works on finding ways to come to an equitable solution to the problems in a relationship. It focuses on the desired goal, rather than on the problems and obstacles involved in achieving that goal. SBT doesn't worry about why you react the way you do; it zeroes in on the way you can change your reactions to achieve harmony in your relationship. In other words, you focus on where you want to be, not how you got to where you are. Life is short. Why waste a precious minute analyzing the past (which you cannot change) when you could be moving toward the situation you desire in your heart? SBT is all about solutions, not assigning blame. SBT therapists don't use long and involved histories in order to find a solution to the problem, so a great deal of time is saved in getting the client moving in the right direction. Wallowing in the

past can be counterproductive and delay the healing that is so badly needed in a relationship. (Many couples don't seek professional help until the last minute. They don't have time for long forays into the past.) The number of therapy sessions in SBT is usually under 10 and averages four to six sessions.

Solution-based therapists and counselors help people analyze times in their lives that are conducive to reaching their desired goals, examine those successes, and strategize on repeating the successful patterns and behaviors in order to move toward the future they envision and desire. This promotes personal change. Based on the work of Dr. Milton H. Erickson, this type of therapy is a positive method of changing a negative situation. Popular author and SBT therapist, Michele Weiner-Davis, M.S.W., has written several books on preventing divorce and how couples can heal their relationships through SBT. (See the Bibliography at the end of this book.)

Weiner-Davis believes that couples should stay together and work through their differences instead of opting for divorce. She points out that divorce doesn't solve the underlying problems and that ways of relating to others will follow each partner into other relationships if the couple divorces. In other words: Divorce doesn't solve anything.

From the beginning of therapy SBT clients learn to set goals so progress can be measured and celebrated. The focus is on where the clients want to go from here and what steps they need to take to get there. Visualizing what they would like the future to be and devising a plan to achieve that goal jumpstarts the change clients want in their relationship. Clients leave with an action plan and the shortest possible route for achieving their goals. SBT focuses on a couple's strengths—the problem-free times in the relationship—keying in on what works and developing a plan to build on that past success. It is assumed that the couple seeking help wants to repair their relationship. The focus is on changes that need to be made for both persons to be happy.

Another key point in SBT is that taking action results in changed behavior and feelings. SBT starts with the question, "What would you like to change?" and progresses from there. When couples leave an SBT session, they have a plan to follow as well as what they should do differently. Small changes are instituted and *that* success builds a foundation for lasting change that saves marriages. (This strategy of making small changes works even if only one partner is making the effort.)

Repeating what worked before to end a dispute or resolve a difference and remembering the old adage,

"If it isn't broken, don't fix it" will move you closer together and help the good times crowd out the negative ones. Deciding what you need to do to get your relationship back on track will involve setting realistic goals and being committed to achieving them. All marriages have problems. No marriage partner is perfect. Certain goals are not possible to achieve. Often the best solutions are the simplest ones. Instead of focusing on the problem, focus on the times your relationship was problem-free. You're looking for small steps in the right direction, not huge makeovers.

<u>Cognitive Behavior Therapy:</u> There are several forms of therapy concentrating on the client's thinking that fall under the heading of cognitive behavior therapy, which is based on the premise that thoughts cause feelings and behaviors; they are not caused by others or things that happen to us. To simplify, the foundation of Cognitive Behavior Therapy (CBT) is built on the concept that the therapist's mandate is to assist clients to improve their thinking and communication, bringing about a better understanding of where the other person is coming from. When people misunderstand others' actions or words the normal response is defensiveness. Cognitive therapists help people improve their communication skills, which, in turn, improve their relationships. CBT gets to the *why*

people react the way they do and it's *that* understanding that clears the way for honest interpretation by following the tried and true axiom of putting one's self in the other person's shoes and understanding what the other person was thinking.

CBT's foundational assumption is that troubles develop when behavior of others is misjudged or misinterpreted. It's the interpretation (misunderstandings, errors in judgment) on the part of the observer (rather than the fault of the one who did or said whatever) that lies at the bottom of the problem between two people.

Our misjudgments or misinterpretations cause us to react in a way that appears irrational so the other person responds in a defensive way and the misunderstanding escalates. CBT therapists guide people in correcting both their thinking and their communication in the hope of aborting future misunderstandings. With couples this plays out in a more accurate interpretation of the other person's statements or actions and paves the way for productive discussion of differences. CBT therapists work to correct distorted thinking.

Solution-Oriented Brief Therapy and Cognitive Behavior Therapy are similar in that neither one resorts to the past to solve today's problems. Both of these therapies are based on the work of Milton

Erickson, the founder of Neuro-Linguistic Programming. Erickson didn't believe in digging up ghosts or rehashing the *he said/she said* conversations *ad nauseum.* Erickson believed that understanding the past was unnecessary to finding a solution to a current problem. SBT and CBT are based on that principle. Both are future-oriented and solution-focused.

CBT helps people be aware of things that might cause them to interpret a situation incorrectly. That technique can change the metabolic activity in the brain (cortex) and alter moods. CBT works from the top down. Cognitive Behavioral Therapy advocates no more than 12 to 15 weeks of treatment.

<u>Imago Relationship Therapy:</u>   At the heart of Imago Relationship Therapy (IRT) is that without change there is no growth and change is the catalyst for healing relationships. Developed by Harville Hendrix, Ph.D., the emphasis is that each partner agrees to change to give the other partner what he or she needs. This flies in the face of the popular idea that people should simply accept others as they are. (See the Bibliography in the back of this book.) In changing to give his or her partner what is needed, a person's own painful experiences are healed—and the partner is healed as well.

Hendrix aptly calls this process *stretching,* and believes that as a person stretches to meet the partner's needs, the person's own needs are met and healing of the relationship takes place. Stretching involves overcoming your own fears and doing the opposite of what you feel like doing: fighting back, arguing, defending yourself. (You know what we're talking about, right?)

The result is that both partners begin to see each other for who they are—fears, dreams, and all. Hendrix calls this a *conscious* relationship, where the cohesiveness of the couple (rather than the two individuals separately) is emphasized and nurtured. The position of the Imago therapist is one of a facilitator and the important thing is the relationship between the two halves of the couple, not the relationship between each half of the couple and the therapist. Imago therapy becomes unnecessary as each partner learns to use its principles in everyday situations. Hendrix advocates what he calls The Conscious Marriage—one that helps a person meet his or her unmet childhood needs in positive ways. Imago Therapy makes the therapist into the facilitator of the couple's healing process, transferring the focus from the therapist to the couple.

Imago Relationship Therapy (IRT) operates from the principle that all things in the universe (including couples) are a whole unit, meaning they are essentially connected, but still able to experience separateness. IRT sees finding a mate and adjusting to marriage is unconsciously attempting to reconnect childhood connections that disconnected. IRT's goal is to help couples reach what Hendrix calls a *conscious* marriage.

Striving for a conscious marriage gets to the root of the power struggle by helping couples isolate and understand any barriers to intimacy, such as unrealistic expectations that no human being could fulfill. Couples in IRT also learn new skills for changing behaviors and how to meet one another's needs. The focus is on compassion, empathy, connection and communion between the partners through a three-part dialogue process germane to IRT. Used consistently the Imago process can transform a rocky relationship to one of spiritual evolution, emotional maturity, and mutual acceptance and healing.

The term *Imago* is Latin for the word *image*. Hendrix chose imago as a name for this therapy because it personifies the type of person one would be seeking to help him or her find the sense of wholeness that was lost in childhood. The search for the ideal mate would gravitate toward the person who best represented the searcher's unconscious image forming in his mind since birth. Based on the qualities evidenced by key people in the searcher's life (mother, father, siblings) the searcher's Imago would evidence both positive and negative traits, with the negative ones sharply defined since that is where the searcher had unfinished business. The imago is both an unconscious image of the opposite sex and an image of the searcher's self. Hendrix believes that a person marries to continue his or her own psychological and emotional growth and not for any altruistic reason. And all of this is unconscious, with the marriage partner getting the blame for all the unhappiness in the marriage.

The goal of IRT is the healing of childhood wounds of *both* partners through a conscious marriage where growth on every level is the goal—in a safe, healthy and whole relationship. (See Bibliography at the end of the book.)

Keys To Understanding

• *Don't give in to your anger and frustration at the immediate situation. Remember how much you love this woman and how much you want the marriage to succeed.*

• *Seek professional help sooner rather than later.*

• *What you want is small steps in the right direction, not huge makeovers.*

• *Improve your communication skills.*

• *Change yourself to give your partner what is needed.*

Author's Note: I highly recommend another therapy that has been very helpful to many. This technique is being used more and more by psychologists and psychiatrists around the country because of its high success rate. Many people just call it tapping, but the technical term is thought field therapy.

TEN:

Using Thought Field Therapy (TFT)

"Elementary my dear Watson."
Basil Rathbone
The Adventures of Sherlock Holmes 1939

Tom, Mary and their two children, Alexa and Jeremiah, are having a hard time dealing with menopause. Even though Mary is the one actually suffering the physical effects, the entire family is being affected by the emotional strain associated with it. Yes, this storm shall pass as they always do, but how can the family maintain emotional strength, stay positive, and actually support Mary while she undergoes this difficult change?

It's no secret that a family dealing with a spouse who's suffering from hormonal imbalance, will deal with emotional distress at some point or another. Any change creates stress, which affects what people think, say and do; and menopause certainly creates a great deal of change. Stress wreaks havoc on relationships, not to mention its effects on the mind and body, which can lead to physical illness and depression.

To overcome this problem, one of the most successful cutting edge methods people can use is a technique borrowed from Energy Psychology called *Thought Field Therapy*. TFT is an incredibly simple method for dealing with stress, which can be used by the ailing spouse to hasten recovery, as well as by the family to overcome difficult times.

<u>TFT Background:</u>   TFT was created in the mid 1970s by three professionals, psychiatrist John Diamond, chiropractor George Goodhardt, and psychologist Roger Callahan. It's a combination of eastern energy therapy and some of the western cognitive therapies included in this book. It's a simple process that literally removes energy blocks at all levels in the body, which helps regain mental and emotional balance.

In essence it's a very powerful technique that helps release the negative emotions and self-sabotaging thought patterns associated with times of stress, and, on the other hand, it can be used to successfully re-condition the mind to perform at optimal levels. In layman's terms it actually re-programs the brain so that the subject does not feel the discomfort associated with a painful situation or memory, and is free to think more clearly and find solutions.

TFT masterfully combines elements of cognitive therapy, acupressure, biofeedback, hypnosis and eye movement desensitization and reprocessing (EMDR).

Once learned it can be practiced individually with great results, and can also be combined by a medical professional with other forms of therapy, as part of a comprehensive medical treatment program.

TFT is applied by using acupressure (repetitive tapping with two fingers), on certain sites of the body (face, chest, underarms and hands), while stating acceptance phrases aimed at transcending a specific problem.

<u>Basic Principles of TFT:</u>   TFT works on a basic principle of self-acceptance, which has been shown to increase emotional balance. This principle states that no matter what the situation, the subject accepts himself or herself, which helps with creativity and emotional resiliency during difficult circumstances.

There is a saying that goes, "What you resist persists. What you accept goes away." This applies to one of the most interesting aspects of TFT, which leads subjects to the acceptance of a specific problem.

The tendency of most people is to run away from problems. This denial gives the problem greater psychological significance which makes things much worse. On the other hand, fighting against the problem also empowers it, and creates even more problems.

The beauty of TFT is that it allows people to face the problem directly, without resistance, and without having to relive the entire painful memory; just enough of it to focus on it, accept it and transcend it as quickly as possible.

The physical tapping, combined with the emotional/mental self-acceptance aspect of the technique, removes blocks within the intricate network of electrical energy pathways called the *meridians*. This *meridian system* distributes energy throughout the body to maintain proper health.

<u>The Thought Field and the Effects of Thoughts and Emotions:</u>   Our bodies are mostly made up of matter, which is dense energy that resonates at low vibrations, which we can actually see with the naked eye.   On the other hand the body also has energy levels referred to as the *thought field*, which resonate at much higher vibrations which we cannot see. This resembles the visible spectrum of light and the non-visible spectrum.

To illustrate this, one can imagine that the body has three interconnected energy levels: physical, mental and emotional. It helps to imagine that feelings (basically comfort or discomfort) are generated by the *emotional body.* These feelings then group themselves into thoughts in the *mental body,* and are ultimately experienced by the *physical body.* Then imagine that these three levels are constantly affecting each other, thus creating the experience of reality.

The effects of thoughts, which are basically energy resonating at higher vibrations than matter, have been studied by many scientists over the years, and recently by Dr. Emoto in Japan, who has proven that thoughts affect the structure of water droplets as they turn into ice crystals. And even more convincing evidence of this is the recent Quantum Physics *Double Slit Experiment* which has shown that thoughts alter matter at the sub-atomic level.

This helps illustrate that whatever affects the mind affects the body, and vice-versa. In other words the effects of thoughts and emotions are not confined to the brain and actually influence the *energy field* within and around the body. This *thought field* is similar to the *ionosphere,* the layer of electromagnetic energy that flows through our planet and surrounds it.

In our bodies it's also known as the *aura* and can be seen through an astonishingly convincing process called Kirlian Photography. Interestingly enough Einstein's E=mc2 formula shows how energy and matter are interchangeable and actually influence each other, which support the basis of energy medicine.

According to eastern philosophy, this energy, which is referred to as Chi, Qi, or Prana, flows through the body's *meridian system,* which happens to correspond with specific sites of the nervous and endocrine systems.

When people experience positive emotional/mental states, this energy flows freely throughout the body. However, when people experience negative emotional states, the energy flow is blocked. This produces a disruption in the system and affects the mind and the body simultaneously, because the negative thoughts and emotions are literally stored within the *thought field* (as well as within the body), in what is known as *cellular memory.*

These disruptions are experienced as muscular stress, tension, irritability, depression, headaches, anxiety, insomnia, physical pain, illness and many other symptoms.

Traditionally, eastern medicine would remove those blocks applying acupuncture needles to hundreds of specific sites within the *meridian system.*

However, TFT uses painless acupressure on only 12 sites and produces similar results. These sites have been selected after years of experience with muscle testing, which has determined that these specific points present the most amount of relief.

<u>Variety of TFT Protocols:</u>   TFT has gained worldwide recognition and support from celebrities such as Deepak Chopra and Cheryl Richardson. Gary Craig has been teaching EFT since 1990 in workshops all over the country, and has reportedly helped thousands of individuals overcome problems such as: Addictions, Allergies, Vision Problems, Headaches, Panic/Anxiety, Asthma, Trauma, PTSD, Abuse, Depression and ADD-ADHD. Gary has created a version of the technique called EFT (Emotional Freedom Technique).Gary maintains a powerful website where practitioners can share information related to specific applications and how to overcome common challenges. The web address is http://www.emofree.com

There are other versions of TFT such as the *Tapas Acupressure Technique* (TAT) and *Energy Diagnostics,* which use slightly different suggestive phrases and acupressure protocols. Since TFT is so flexible, many new versions are appearing as therapists become more specialized.

What practitioners such as Gary Craig have done, is to adapt old techniques to the current understanding of modern energy medicine and have added powerful physiological tools to help release blocks at the emotional, mental and physical levels, thus yielding faster results than any other therapy to date.

In their book, <u>Instant Emotional Healing</u>, Dr. George Pratt and Dr. Peter Lambrou, two respected psychologists from California, state that they have successfully treated 18,000 patients using their own very comprehensive and highly effective version of TFT, called *Emotional Self Mastery* (ESM). Their scientifically supported book is an invaluable source of background information on TFT and offers very detailed protocols for dealing with a variety of issues. It also includes a complete section on performance enhancement which can be used after removing negative blocks in order to condition the mind for greater success in sports, work and family life.

<u>Length of Treatment with TFT:</u>   Any form of TFT uses the same basic methodology and only takes five to ten minutes to apply. The catch is that it is problem-specific, which means that it deals with one problem or one aspect of a problem at a time.

This is because the brain stores thoughts and feelings the same way the *thought field* does. Each neuron stores a part of a given memory (thoughts and feelings) and is physically linked to other neurons that hold other memories, making up an incredibly vast number of connections called the *neural network.*

This understanding is crucial, because as TFT treats a specific emotion, a person may notice that the discomfort he or she is working on is linked to many other memories, mimicking the neural connections. In TFT each of these must be addressed independently.

This process can be compared to pealing away the layers of an onion, since memories are stored in layers. TFT works by quickly peeling layer after layer, until minimal or no emotional pain is present, which then allows the subject to deal with the situation without an emotional block.

Each layer may take five to ten minutes to treat, but if the problem is complicated, it may take several months to reach the desired results. If this is the case enlisting the help of an experienced practitioner would be very helpful, especially since people may tap into painful sub-conscious layers that may temporarily throw them off track without the appropriate support.

<u>Practical Use of EFT:</u>   Let's choose EFT as an example of how TFT works, simply because of its simplicity and because it illustrates how most variations work. For more information on specific EFT applications, including tapping site diagrams, visit http://www.eflexx.com.

The entire EFT procedure for overcoming distressful emotions includes the following steps:

1. Select a specific Emotional Discomfort to work on
2. Determine SUDS
3. Create a Mental Movie of the Distressful Situation
4. Recite a Setup Phrase
5. Apply Initial Tapping Sequence
6. Apply Bridge for the first time
7. Determine Second SUDS
8. Apply Secondary Tapping Sequence
9. Apply Bridge a second time
10. Determine SUDS
11. Apply Eye Roll

Let's use Tom, from the story mentioned earlier, to illustrate the application of EFT protocols.

Tom is frustrated because of his wife's erratic behavior. He wants to help, but feels overwhelmed by the whole ordeal. The first thing Tom does, is find a comfortable, quiet place to sit, closes his eyes, and decides to work on frustration, because this is the most upsetting aspect for him.

He then establishes a subjective point of reference, where he rates how much psychological discomfort he feels on a 0 to10 scale called SUDS (Subjective Units of Disturbance Scale). He does this before, during and after the procedure to notice his own progress. Initially he determines that he's an eight on the scale.

The next thing Tom does, is that he keeps his eyes closed and creates a mental movie of his distressful situation, where he visualizes for a couple of minutes the sequence of events that led to his frustration. He makes sure to be as specific as possible and only focuses on the situation at hand, instead of also thinking about having to go grocery shopping, for example.

He then continues with a Setup Phrase, where he uses one hand to tap repetitively on the fleshy part of the other hand, known as the Karate Chop Point, while stating the following phase: "I deeply and completely accept myself, even though I'm frustrated with Mary's attitude towards me." He knows that the more focused he gets, the more effective the technique will be, so he repeats this phrase at least three times while tapping the spot and focusing on the mental movie he created earlier.

Tom then opens his eyes and proceeds with the initial tapping sequence on the 12 meridian sites associated with EFT. Since the body has two sides and the meridian system has the same points on each, he knows that he can tap on either the left or right side of his body. While mentally repeating "This Problem!"

Tom uses two fingers to tap repeatedly on each of the following sites for about five seconds:

1. Corner of the eyebrow next to the bridge of the nose
2. Outside corner of the eye
3. Under the eye
4. Under the nose
5. Under the lower lip
6. Under the arm (near the armpit)
7. Collarbone (near the sternum)
8. Outer corner of the base of the thumbnail
9. Outer corner of the base of the index fingernail
10. Outer corner of the base of the middle finger nail
11. Outer corner of the base of the little fingernail
12. Gamut Point located on the back of the hand, between the bones of the little finger and the ring finger.

After this initial sequence which takes about one minute, Tom proceeds with what is called The Bridge. Tom knows that what's affecting him is the emotion associated with the mental picture, so he's going to engage his sense of sight along with the left and right sides of his brain in order to scramble the negative feeling and be able to release the emotional ties. This part of EFT includes a powerful technique used to treat Post Traumatic Stress Disorder called *eye movement desensitization reprocessing,* EMDR for short.

He does this by continuing to tap on the Gamut Point while still focusing on the problem as he did during the tapping sequence. He then closes his eyes, while continuing to tap, then, while keeping his head perfectly straight and without moving it, he opens his eyes, looks straight down and to the right and proceeds to trace an imaginary circle around his face, moving his eyes slowly from right to left, then immediately in the opposite direction. This takes him about three to four seconds.

While still tapping on the Gamut Point, he hums about five notes (from the happy birthday song for example), which engages the right side of his brain related to art, then counts from one to five, to engage the left side of his brain, which deals with logic. This takes him less than five seconds and he continues tapping on the Gamut Point for another 30 seconds.

Tom then checks his SUDS again and notices that he's magically at a 3-4 on the scale.

He's done with the first sequence! Even though he feels a sense of release, Tom knows he can do better, so he goes for a second round. This time, he does not have to create the mental movie again; all he needs to do is focus on the remaining discomfort while stating the setup phrase slightly differently: "I deeply and completely accept myself, even though I STILL feel a bit frustrated with Mary."

He then proceeds to tap on all points and when he gets to the hand, he declares the following phrase a couple of times while tapping on each of the fingers, "I release this frustration for my own benefit." He continues with the second bridge and then rechecks his SUDS.

At this point, he tries to focus on how he feels and notices that the frustration is gone completely, which means the EFT procedure has worked. If it had not worked, Tom knows he could have continued with several tapping sequences until his SUDS reached 0.

Because he's feeling a sense of release from the frustration, he decides to seal off the procedure by doing what's called the Eye Roll, which engages his brain in different ways, and further enhances the mental reconditioning he so desperately needed.

He does this by simply closing his eyes, right after checking his SUDS, while keeping his head perfectly straight again, without moving it, and then opening his eyes, looking straight down towards his feet and then letting his eyes follow an imaginary line across the floor in front of him, which then goes up to the sky and ends directly above his head.

After this sequence, which took only five to ten minutes, Tom feels emotionally stronger and has even started getting ideas about how to solve the problem.

<u>Final Note on TFT:</u> Now that Tom knows all about managing his emotions with TFT, he can show his family how to apply this marvelous technique and help Mary get back on track even while going through menopause. The great news is that this once painful experience can become an opportunity for growth for the entire family and may even lead to a greater sense of fulfillment, since emotional blocks no longer have to be an issue.

Even if Tom and Mary's relationship does not survive the menopause storm, TFT has helped them realize that they do not have to be victims to painful memories, and that they are free to decide to plant seeds of hope for a much better future for themselves and everyone around them.

This chapter was contributed by Mike Angulo, Life Coach. Mike can be reached at http://www.Eflexx.com.

PART THREE
TAKING CARE

ELEVEN:

Forgiveness

"Love means never having to say you're sorry."
Ali MacGraw
Love Story 1970

No, you didn't deserve what has happened to your marriage because of your wife's hormone imbalance. Neither did she deserve it. But here you are in the middle of one of the most frustrating battles of your adult life and, if you'll be honest, you hate it. And there's no one person or event you can blame.

You cannot change the past. You cannot just make the situation go away. But there is one simple little technique you *can* do all by yourself to make everything you're both going through a little easier. Try forgiveness.

If you are harboring unforgiveness toward anyone, you are stuck in an emotional prison. You are the one who suffers the most, not the person or the situation you are angry about. Many times the other person you are not forgiving doesn't even know you're angry, so it's of no consequence to him or her if you continue to stay in an unforgiving mode. It's in everyone's best interest that you choose to forgive.

Forgive your wife. Forgive yourself. Forgive God for letting this happen. And while you're at it, liberate yourself completely by forgiving anyone who has either intentionally or unintentionally hurt you. When you forgive, you're not excusing what the other person did (or didn't do). Forgiveness erases the uncollected debt of apology that you are owed and frees you to be forgiven by others that you have either intentionally or unintentionally hurt. (No, you are not without blame! All human beings mess up at some point and need forgiveness.) You have two choices: choose to hang onto the hurts of the past and prevent healing from taking place in your marriage, or choose to forgive and release the hurts and enable yourself to move forward. Don't worry about retribution or revenge or getting even. What goes around comes around and anger is your enemy. Holding onto anger gives you the illusion of control over the relationship because the other person needs your forgiveness (whether they know they need it or not). Your concern is to keep short accounts in your own heart and mind when it comes to offenses, whether you offend someone and have to apologize or someone has offended you.

Once you've truly forgiven someone, don't bring the offense up again. This frees you to concentrate on the really important things in life, such as constructively rebuilding your relationship with those you love. There have been many studies documenting that both emotional and physical health improve when a person truly forgives another person.

Forgiving someone doesn't mean you won't be hurt again. People being people, if your home is under the mantle of menopause, things can escalate very quickly. What begins as a simple statement by one partner can become a major battlefield. Most logical disagreements are really about fear and shame. Here's an example. Sara says, "It's cold in here." John says, "How can you say that? It's 75 degrees!"

Sara could have said, "I'm *feeling* cold." That's a whole different thing from the temperature in the house being cold. But she didn't say it that way. And no matter if that is what she really meant, John is going to see it as a failure on his part to provide heat for his wife because he feels he doesn't seem to be able to do anything right these days.

John is not addressing her point at all, and Sara is not expressing what she really means. Far from a logical analysis of the relationship between sensation and temperature, John's remark is completely reactive. He was neither thinking nor listening. He simply responded in a knee-jerk fashion. His reaction was meant to devalue an opinion that he found threatening. Naturally Sara is going to react to his remark. She now feels he doesn't value her, which raises her anxiety. They both feel devalued by the other, even though no one is trying to devalue anybody. They are trying to avoid the discomfort of their own underlying fear and shame. All of this is unconscious. All they know is they are angry with each other.

The fact that it is 75 degrees in the room neither supports nor contradicts Sara's sensation of being cold. Their statements provide different bits of information, with their own unique contributions to the discussion. Couples make a terrible mistake when they think one kind of response, be it mostly logical or mostly emotional, is superior to the other. In reality they are different dimensions, each important in its own right.

So when couples have disputes about bills—*We don't have any money. I can't pay the bills.*—or the temperature—*It's cold in here.*—the basis of the remarks is powered by a woman's fear of deprivation and isolation and by a man's fear of failing as a provider—not by any difference in reasoning.

Much of the resentment that occurs in relationships is not about material differences; it's about the perception that your emotions are controlled, if not manipulated, by your partner. He makes her anxious; she makes him feel like a failure.

If this is the syndrome you're caught in, consider the role of serotonin in keeping things on an even keel. Serotonin is a neurotransmitter in the central nervous system. When serotonin levels are normal it's easier to control your reactions. It's also easier to let go of anger and negative thoughts. When your serotonin levels are low, however, you are anxious and react more negatively. Your outlook is gloomy; you obsess about negative events; you are more prone to anger and irritability, and you can fall quickly into fear and shame.

Forgiveness in a marriage is no simple matter. Both people are involved in the problem. (No one has a problem alone.) Neither partner is solely responsible for any problem that arises in a marriage. Nor is either partner solely innocent. The balance may be 80/20, but each partner bears some of the responsibility. Both the righteous anger and the defensive anger must be surrendered in order to have a state of forgiveness so the marriage can begin to heal. True forgiveness includes reconciliation—a term that means mutual openness and mutual willingness to make changes for the sake of the relationship. A willingness to forgive requires each person's admitting he or she is partly responsible for the problem. This requires both honesty and humility. This is the point on which a lot of potential forgiveness and reconciliation gets hung up. Both people must be willing to admit partial blame and be willing to make changes that will allow mutual healing.

When one of the people involved is a woman dealing with menopause, forgiveness may not be possible until a later date, if ever. The reason is that during menopause the limbic system (the parts of the brain that store and process memories and emotion), is constantly being stimulated due to the hormonal upheaval in a woman's system and also due to the rewiring that takes place. The hypothalamus, in particular, controls strong emotions such as sadness, anger, and painful memories, that (along with self-reflection and introspection) take center stage. (See chapter two.) This is the time that bad memories from ten, twenty or more years earlier pop into the brain and out of the mouth. The unsuspecting husband may not even remember some of the incidents his wife is bringing up. Emotional wounds that have been festering inside all those years will erupt into a list that amazes both the husband and the wife, leaving them both wondering where this is all coming from. This is also the time that spiritual renewal and reflection play a bigger role in the menopausal woman's life. (Perhaps this is the first time in her adult life that the woman has had the time to even think of these things?)

Along with all this introspection comes the deep need for forgiveness. No relationship can survive without forgiveness—of ourselves, of our mates, our parents, our children, our families, our friends, and perfect strangers—and even God (if we don't know whom else to blame), for allowing certain out-of-our-control things to happen.

Forgiveness is not the same as forgetting. When you forgive someone you cancel a debt that person owes you (whether they know they owe it or not). When you forgive you also give up the right to ever bring up the thing the other person did and you give up the right to ever use it against them in any way. What if the offense keeps popping back into your mind? When that happens, true forgiveness refuses to think about it or dwell on it, putting it out of the mind deliberately. What a person thinks about evokes emotions, which, in turn, stimulate biochemical reactions in our bodies. Unforgiveness can wreak havoc with your mental (and physical) health.

Forgiving God may seem spiritually incorrect, but there are times when God is the only one big enough to shoulder the blame for something horrific that has happened, such as a natural disaster that claims hundreds of lives. If you have been holding

God accountable for something that was a disaster in *your* life, letting go of the hurt and resentment is a healthy thing for you to do, and God is big enough to take it.

What if you are the one who needs to be forgiven? There is an art to asking for forgiveness. Saying I'm sorry is not the best way to go because it almost sounds trite or overused and the person you are apologizing to does not have to respond. The best way is to ask, "Will you forgive me?" The other person must answer your question—one way or the other. Neither one of you is perfect. You have both made mistakes and will make more. It may take time to work through hurts that have been building up in your relationship, but persistence will pay off. Your marriage is worth the effort.

What about those women who undergo a hysterectomy and experience *surgical menopause?* The same emphasis on past hurts that need forgiveness, periods of great introspection, the resurfacing of bad memories and brain-rewiring all happen to women who have hysterectomies. Usually it just happens at a younger age than natural menopause.

Forgiveness is not a one-time event. It's an ongoing process we all must participate in so that we can live healthy, productive and satisfying lives. To forgive without reservation is to free one's self for the best that life has to offer. It's not easy to forgive someone who has hurt you, but the rewards of forgiveness are long-lasting and far-reaching, affecting not only you, but all whose lives you touch. Take responsibility and forgive daily—hourly, if necessary—to reap the benefits of a healthier mindset and better physical health.

Keys to Understanding

• *Try forgiveness and get out of your emotional prison.*

• *Don't bring offenses up again after you have forgiven them (or been forgiven for them). This allows you to concentrate on rebuilding your relationship.*

• *True forgiveness includes reconciliation—a term that means mutual openness and mutual willingness to make changes for the sake of the relationship.*

• *Don't say, I'm sorry. It's been used so much it might not ring true. The best way to ask forgiveness is to say, Will you forgive me? This forces an answer, either yes or no.*

• *Forgiveness is not a one-time event.*

TWELVE:

Which Hormones Do What?

"We all go a little mad sometimes."
Anthony Perkins
Psycho 1960

A woman can be in good health according to medical assessment and lab-work and still feel terrible. She can go to numerous doctors and specialists and alternative practitioners and still not get to the bottom line explanation of why she feels unwell. Typical comments from the medical world range from *there's nothing wrong with you,* to *let's do more tests to see if we can get to the bottom of this.* Neither response helps her get back to normal.

The thing that will help her the most is getting her hormones balanced. Hormones are the messengers that tell the body what is needed and where. Each hormone has a specific mission. *Melatonin,* for example, regulates the biological clock and helps maintain regular sleep patterns. *ADH* (antidiuretic hormone) maintains fluid and electrolyte balance in the kidneys. *LH* (luteinizing hormone) notifies the ovaries to produce estrogens and begin ovulation in women. *FSH* (follicle stimulating hormone) helps with the maturing of ovarian follicles. *ACTH* (adreno-corticotrophic hormone) stimulates the adrenal gland to produce cortisol. *HGH* (human growth hormone) helps tissue growth in many areas of the body. *PRL* (prolactin) is the hormone that lets a woman's milk drop down for lactation. *MSH* (melanocyt) works on skin tone. TSH,T3 and T4 are hormones related to thyroid function. *TSH* (thyroid stimulating hormone), *T3* (triiodothyronine) and *T4* (thyroxine) are all generated in the thyroid gland. *TSH* is involved in cortisol production, *T3* and *T4* have to do with the development of the brain and reproductive tract as well as regulating metabolism.

Insulin regulates blood sugar levels. *Cortisol* is involved in response to stress and immune suppression. *DHEA* (dehydroepiandrosterone) stimulates the immune system, promotes a better resistance to stress, helps keep the skin flexible, improves bone tissue and can increase libido. It is the precursor to the production of several other hormones. *Estradiol, estrone* and *estriol* (the estrogens) help maintain elasticity in connective tissue, preserve bone mass and promote vascular health. *Pregnenelone* repairs brain and nerve tissue, works on aging skin and increases energy and mobility as well as reducing the effects of stress. *Progesterone* prepares and maintains the lining of the uterus for pregnancy. *Testosterone* is the precursor for estrogen, meaning it triggers the production of progesterone. It also works on the libido, maintains muscle strength and tone, decreases body fat and promotes confidence.

Natural hormones that are precisely identical to the molecular structure of hormones produced in the human body are the only hormones many doctors recommend for their patients. Made from yams and soybeans, they can work wonders in a woman's body that has been depleted of sufficient hormone levels due to perimenopause and/or menopause.

Reported results from various doctors using bioidentical hormone replacement therapy for their patients include better memory and less brain-fog, more stamina, less PMS, younger-looking skin, fewer mood swings, better sleep, better sex, better weight control, less anxiety and less depression.

Timing of bioidentical hormone replacement therapy is important. If the body becomes deficient in a hormone, waiting too long to supplement may mean the resulting signs in the body (wrinkles, for example), may be unable to be reversed.

Conventional medical schools do not prepare their graduates in the area of natural hormones. In addition many medical schools are underwritten by the large pharmaceutical companies, who provide multitudes of samples of their products and train the doctors in prescribing them. These are not natural (bioidentical) hormones but are chemical formulas that can be patented. (Translation: Synthetic hormones produce income for the company every time a prescription is filled.) Synthetic hormones do not usually allow the patient to achieve total hormonal balance.

Bioidentical hormone replacement therapy certainly cannot guarantee that the recipient has discovered the fountain of youth, but a degree of youthfulness can be restored and enjoyed.

Most conventional substitute hormones have a different chemical structure from the hormones the human body produces. This major difference aggravates imbalances already in existence in the body.

Unless a hormone prescription is a precise replica of the natural hormone found in the human body, it's likely to cause more problems than it helps. Take estrogen replacement for example. If a woman is taking the normally prescribed conjugated equine estrogen (made from the urine of pregnant horses), she is introducing a foreign substance into her body. No wonder it causes problems! The presence of CEE (conjugated equine estrogen) in the body makes standard blood tests measuring estrogen levels basically worthless. It takes at least two months after stopping CEE for the synthetic estrogen to leave the body.

Achieving hormonal balance is not a one-time event. It can take several months before a course of bioidentical hormone replacement therapy will make a change in hormone levels. So achieving balance is an ongoing process. It takes information and education, commitment and time to restore healthy balance to the levels of hormones in the body. But the rewards are very much worth the effort.

Bioidentical hormone therapy can turn back the biological clock, giving a woman more energy, mental clarity, renewed sensuality, and a positive outlook on life. Why put chemical synthetic hormone substitutes into the body when it's just as easy to take precise replicas of the hormones the body produces naturally?

Keys To Understanding

• *What will help her the most is getting her hormones balanced.*

• *Use precisely identical natural hormones, not synthetic ones.*

• *Using synthetic hormones is likely to cause more problems than it helps.*

• *Achieving hormonal balance is not a one-time event. It's an ongoing process.*

• *It makes sense to take precise replicas of the body's natural hormones.*

THIRTEEN:

Natural Supplements Can Help You Both

"May the force be with you."
Harrison Ford
Star Wars 1977

Dealing with your partner's menopausal symptoms and trying to save your marriage are going to be very hard on your physical body. The stress can become almost unbearable. There will probably be times when the stress is so bad you simply feel like hanging it all up either by jumping into your pool never to leave it, or sitting in your car with the garage door shut and the windows open with the engine running.

Most of us never reach the state where we take such disastrous action but the very idea that we are thinking about it shows that our bodies and minds are extremely stressed. The fact that we want to end our suffering by such drastic action should tell us that we need to do something and we need to do it quickly.

Relieving stress, anxiety and depression isn't easy. Usually when you tell your doctor about how you are feeling he takes out his prescription pad and writes you a prescription for something like Prozac, Paxil or a generic form of Xanax. All of these are anti-depressants/anti-anxiety drugs.

Doctors usually recommend a class of drugs known as benzodiazepines which include drugs like Xanax, Valium and Ativan. These drugs are supposed to take the edge off by targeting GABA receptor sites. In addition to being an amino acid that you can buy from your local health food store, GABA is also one of the central nervous system's most important neuro-transmitters. What GABA does is directly stimulate receptors that inhibit (or calm down) activity in your overactive brain. When your brain is hyperactive during a marital crisis or your response to one of your partner's menopausal symptoms, it needs to be calmed down so you can better focus. GABA helps calm you down. It helps make you less anxious or less irritable. In effect it helps you to better deal with the stressful situations you are going through. It helps you control your reactions. When you feel overwhelmed, when you feel like your heart is beating a hundred times a minute, you need to relax and calm down. GABA can help you do that.

GABA is safe, non-toxic and the good thing about it is that it's not habit-forming. Once you are on something like Xanax or Paxil it is extremely difficult to get off it. Products like Xanax also target the GABA receptor sites but the similarities end there. Benzodiazepines also have a negative effect on the central nervous system. They are also habit-forming and hypnotic. The drugs can make sleeping difficult and even lead to cognitive problems. They also can make you a bit wobbly. A study conducted years ago linked at least 10,000 hip fractures per year to these drugs. They also could affect your driving ability and certainly are suspect in thousands of automobile accidents annually.

Benzodiazepines are especially risky for older people as they have much less ability to overcome the drugs' negative side effects. Their bodies are much more sensitive to the actions of these drugs. And these drugs are very addictive. Although these prescriptions are usually written for short-term use, patients can end up dependent on them for years. In a 2007 study from Columbia University it has been estimated that nearly 20% of older Americans are taking these drugs.

The other problem is that anxiety itself isn't really a disease. Sometimes it is very normal to feel anxious. In fact, a little stress makes us more alert and can give us an edge in certain situations. The problem is when the stress or anxiety becomes debilitating and prevents us from leading normal lives.

If you are suffering from anxiety you should take a hard look at GABA. A 500 mg. capsule three times per day might help calm you down so you can get through this stressful life experience. For quick release during a bad anxiety attack simply open a capsule and pour the contents into a glass of water and stir.

<u>Other Possible Supplements:</u>   There are a number of other possible supplements that you should look into besides GABA. L-Theanine is an amino acid that is found in green tea. L-Theanine helps raise your body's own levels of GABA and also slows down alpha-wave activity in your brain. The product 5-HTP is also an amino acid supplement. 5-HTP helps boost levels of serotonin which is a neurotransmitter that is involved in mood and sleep. The drug Paxil is one of a class of drugs known as *serotonin uptake inhibitors* but Paxil is very habit-forming and has numerous side effects including sexual dysfunction. So 5-HTP can help boost serotonin levels as Paxil does, but without all the side effects.

If your mind is racing when you try to get to sleep you can always reach for the Lunesta prescription but, while it will put you to sleep, it is also something you could become dependent on and that is also very hypnotic. Some people have done things that they simply don't remember after falling asleep with Lunesta.

Some natural sleep aids would be Valerian which is an anxiety-reducing herb that should be taken at bedtime and could help you sleep. Melatonin is also something that might help with sleep. So a combination of Valerian, 5-HTP and Melatonin could be a good combination before bedtime. Dosages would be 3 mg. of Melatonin, 50 mg. of 5-HTP, 200 mg. of Valerian and 500 mg. of GABA. Some people just take a higher dose of melatonin. For instance, best-selling author, Suzanne Somers, in her new book, *Breakthrough*, mentions that she takes 20mg of melatonin each night before bed, which helps her to achieve 8-9 hours of sleep each night.

You might want to research a new product called Mellow-Tone, a proprietary blend that includes melatonin which is delivered via strips placed on the tongue, leading to a greater absorption of the melatonin to the body.

Another low cost natural sleep aid is New Health Corp's, Amazing Sleep Plus, (www.amazingsleepplus.com), which is a proprietary formula of 5-HTP, melatonin, Gaba, valerian and other products.

<u>What If You Are Now Becoming Depressed?</u>   If you are being rejected by your wife and sex has been non-existent for weeks (or even months), you are probably going to be down on yourself. There are two things to remember here: You shouldn't let another person define your self-esteem and you may need something to help you get through this.

There are, of course, the various pharmaceutical anti-depressants such as Prozac. But these are addictive and often come with various side effects. Therapy, especially EFT (Emotional Freedom Technique), can help but you may also need a mood elevator or two.

There have been numerous clinical studies conducted on the benefits or non-benefits of St. John's Wort. Several studies have shown it to be as effective as antidepressant drugs in dealing with mild or moderate depression. In fact the herb is often recommended in Europe instead of drugs. Other studies, including a major National Institute of Health study that focused on moderate to severe depression, showed no improvements with St. John's Wort. I think the key here is the severity of the depression. If things are so bad you are contemplating suicide, then you probably need something stronger than St. John's Wort as well as some serious counseling. If, however, you have a bad case of the blahs and are feeling down on yourself, taking a capsule of St. John's Wort three times a day might help you out. As far as the dosage is concerned, probably 400 mg. three times a day would do the trick, although the British Herbal Medicine Association Scientific Committee in 1983 suggested much higher dosages in the range of 2-4 grams three times a day would be acceptable.

The exact way in which St. John's Wort works is unclear but it seems to involve the inhibition of serotonin (5-HTP) re-uptake, much like the conventional selective serotonin reuptake inhibitors (SSRI) antidepressants like Prozac and Paxil.

St. John's Wort may react negatively with other drugs, so if you are taking other drugs, especially those for epilepsy or other immunosuppressant problems, or if you are taking any benzodiazepines, you should discuss this product with your primary care physician before taking it. If you want to try and stay away from drugs you may want to try the above herbs and amino acids. They have proven to be very effective for some men who are dealing with anxiety, sleeping problems and mild to moderate depression.

There are, of course, other products that you probably should be taking while you are going through this crisis. A good multi-vitamin is a necessity. A good pharmaceutical-grade fish oil helps with inflammation and mood and is probably next in line after your multivitamin. There is also a new product that you might want to take a look at: stem cell nutrition.

Unfortunately when the body is going through a lot of stress the immune system has to suffer. Your adrenals are on overload and stress taxes everything from your heart to your aching back. You may develop chest palpitations or nervous body twitches. This is simply your body trying to tell you that it needs some help.

The latest development in nutraceuticals is stem cell nutrition.

Since you were born your body has produced stem cells to help you grow and heal. Your own bone marrow is the source of all the stem cells you need unless you suffer from a medical emergency. Here is basically how it works:

You cut yourself. A message from the cut site is sent to the bone marrow where the bone marrow releases whatever stem cells are needed. The stem cells in the blood stream multiply and migrate to the cut site. At the cut site they multiply further and produce tissue to replace the injured tissue. Stem cells have the power to create new brain tissue, new liver tissue, new kidney tissue, new skin tissue, new heart tissue, as well as other types. This is why so many people are traveling overseas to have injections of stem cells.

The Journal of Medical Hypothesis in 2002 postulated that the potential for stem cells in battling degenerative diseases is significant. This has since been confirmed and validated in over 70 known human conditions.

Every stem cell has the ability to become thousands of specific tissue cells.

What if there was a product that could help your body generate its own additional stem cells? Actually there is such a product.

There have been a number of studies that describe the benefits of *aphanizmenon flos aquae* better known as AFA which is the first protein and most ancient food on earth. At the bottom of the food chain, it is the most nutrient-rich food (ounce for ounce) known to be created by nature.

Recently a couple of progressive companies have learned that a couple extracts of AFA could hold tremendous benefits.

It has been shown that ingestion of as little as one gram of these AFA extracts per day increased stem cell production of the bone marrow anywhere from 25-30% within one hour. A 25% increase is the equivalent of up to 3 to 4 million additional stem cells per day.

When your body is undergoing stress and your immune system is compromised you need all the help you can get. There is a company that has taken whole AFA and added a couple of key extracts of AFA which amplify the effect of AFA. The name of the company is Emergent Health Corporation, a publicly traded company. The product they have that stimulates stem cell growth is called *Vita-Stim* (www.vita-stim.com). This product could be a solid addition to your list of supplements. This product could help improve mood, give you more stamina to get through the day and potentially help you in several other areas. The problems that your body is enduring may not become known until your marital situation has been resolved. The key is trying to keep your body as healthy as you possibly can while you are going through this difficult experience.

Where women are concerned, added estrogen can stimulate the hypothalamus gland to release endorphins, with the result that a woman feels better. Recent research has begun to show many more connections between neurochemicals and human moods, such as the links between dopamine and the feeling of joy; between serotonin and sadness; between acetycholine and angst. Recent research has also suggested that low estrogen levels might cause the synapses between cells in the brain to function at a diminished capacity. (Synapses are the spaces between neurons or nerve cells that allow messages to be transferred from one cell to another.) Estrogen might assist this message transfer. Lower levels of estrogen in the brain might, therefore, contribute to the loss of reasoning power and short-term memory loss that some women experience during menopause.

There is no question that you and your wife are both going through a very difficult time. The stress load is huge on both of you. Anything you can do to ease your stress would be a good move. Right now you both need all the help you can get.

Keys To Understanding

• *Know that benzodiazepines have a negative effect on the central nervous system, are habit-forming and hypnotic, can make sleeping difficult, leave you wobbly and could lead to cognitive problems.*

• *Try natural remedies to calm you down rather than pharmaceutical antidepressants.*

• *Some natural supplements such as St. John's Wort may react negatively with pharmaceutical drugs.*

• *Don't let another person define your self-esteem.*

• *Do what you can to ease the stress load on both you and your wife.*

FOURTEEN:

Maybe Your Wife Needs A Vacation

"What we've got here is a failure to communicate."
Strother Martin
Cool Hand Luke 1967

Many couples break up unnecessarily. The thinking is that if things aren't perfect, let's just end the marriage. There is no interest in counseling. And they head off to divorce court to become yet another statistic.

As we have mentioned throughout this book, there are many things happening to the middle-age woman over which she has little control. This can make a woman feel that the only way to end her inner turmoil is to walk away from the marriage. What she may really need is some space to find herself. After years of taking care of her husband and children and with all the changes taking place in her physical and emotional health, she may simply no longer know who she is as a person. The easiest (and least acceptable) answer may seem to be to break up the family, end the marriage and move on. But perhaps if her husband and family could just give her some time and space to work through her issues, she could regain her balance and perspective. Maybe instead of a divorce she just needs a long vacation.

There is a great series of books written by Joan Anderson that deal with this subject. Her first book was the bestseller *A Year By The Sea*. After years of focusing on the needs of others as a wife and mother, Joan was faced with a decision when her husband suddenly announced they had to move to another city for a position he had accepted. Joan decided not to move with her husband and decided instead to move to a family cottage on Cape Cod where she spent an entire year discovering who she was as a person and becoming comfortable with her unique individuality.

She and her husband eventually got back together again and Joan has used her experience to help other women. She gives workshops and seminars that encourage women to take a sabbatical—a period of rest. She reasoned that if college professors can take a sabbatical every seven years to do research, write a book or simply recharge their batteries, why can't wives do it, too?

As women move into the menopausal years the need to step back and refocus is even greater as biological changes actually force introspection. After years of nurturing others perhaps they need some time to nurture themselves. Perhaps they need some time to discover who they are besides someone's wife or mother. It's like Joan Anderson says in her book *A Weekend To Change Your Life* most women in their thirties to their seventies are asking themselves the same question: "After being all things to all people, how can I become what I need to be for myself?"

This is a difficult question to which many women never seem to find the answer. By default they simply continue to exist in a relationship that doesn't meet their needs. Other women simply say to themselves that they want and need a change and opt for the quickest way out: divorce.

What if there were ways to take some time off and have that time respected by the husband? What if there were ways for the woman to learn more about herself? What if there were ways to gain wisdom and a better understanding of who she is as a person without ending the marriage or breaking up the family. Wouldn't that make more sense?

No marriage is perfect and none of us is perfect. There is always someone better somewhere. There is always someone prettier or someone wealthier. If we are looking for perfection in our relationships, we will never find it. If we are looking for perfection in ourselves, we will never find it. Can we learn more about ourselves and still honor the commitment we made to our spouses? The answer is yes.

Every person should examine his or her life and relationships periodically. This becomes both a natural reaction as well as a necessity for most women as they approach middle age and menopause. At this time in their lives women need space. If it isn't available to them in their home or their relationship they will seek it elsewhere.

The idea of a sabbatical makes a lot of sense. With the blessing of an understanding spouse, the woman departs to the destination of her choice to discover who she really is. It could be as short as two weeks, or as long as a year.

Some women feel the need to be absolutely alone during this time. Two weeks or a month totally alone at a seashore cottage in a different part of the country may be perfect for some women, but others may feel the need for the companionship of another woman or two who are also experiencing the same upsets of menopause.

It's hard for men to understand what in the world a woman would do by herself (or with a couple of friends) for two weeks. The fact is that men like their time with other men as well with no women around, and they need it just as much as women need time with other women with no men around. Freedom is a wonderful word for women who are enduring physical, emotional and spiritual changes all at the same time. Getting away from everything and everyone sounds to them like pure heaven on earth.

It's easy for a man to feel rejected if his wife wants to go away without him. But if he truly loves his wife and wants to help her through this difficult time, he will not only grant her his blessing in this sabbatical but also give her a little going-away present (such as a new outfit, or a gift certificate to buy something she chooses herself). It's also important for the man to not come across as needy while she's preparing for her great escape. She doesn't want to feel guilty about needing this time alone. The truth is, she really *does* need it.

Women need this time away from the pressures of home and present relationships to rediscover themselves and reactivate their dreams. As they get older they start wanting more or different things from their relationships and their lives. They are changing and growing and, if their husbands change and grow with them, they can rekindle their relationship and even take it to a higher level.

If the husband resists or denies this need exists, the wife will pull away even farther and faster. If you are a husband who wants to save his marriage, this is the time to give your wife the space she desperately needs to find out who she really is and what she wants in the next phase of her life.

A sabbatical may be just what the doctor *didn't* order.

Keys To Understanding

• *Middle-aged women are experiencing many things over which they have little control.*

• *Giving your wife time and space to rediscover herself may well be the most loving thing you can do for her.*

• *Taking a vacation could help your wife gain wisdom and a better understanding of who she is as a person.*

• *If you are a husband who wants to save his marriage, this is the time to give your wife the space she desperately needs away from the pressures of home and present relationships.*

• *Taking a sabbatical may be exactly what the doctor didn't order.*

FIFTEEN:

What If....? (The Best and Worst Outcomes)

"It's amazing Molly. The love inside, you take it with you."
Patrick Swayze
Ghost 1990

Nearly everything in life is negotiable, including the marriage contract. There is the natural give and take between two people that makes up everyday life. And then there is the hard stuff that surfaces when various forces threaten to tear a couple apart. Conflict happens. Getting to the heart of the matter so the two of you can agree to a compromise and get on with life is made even more difficult if you have different styles of resolving problems. One of you may be someone who problem-solves by talking things out (sometimes in great detail) and the other of you may be someone who would choose to not have the conversation at all but just wait and see how it all works itself out.

What if you do everything right and it doesn't work?

No one can tell you when you should give up on saving your marriage, but if, in spite of everything you've tried, you find yourself heading for divorce court, take a deep breath and try harder *one more time.* Here are some factors you should consider:

Divorce doesn't really *solve* anything. Instead of dealing with the problems, divorce buries them. Wives who walk away from their marriages are assuming someone else is to blame for their unhappiness and discontent. When people divorce they take their unsolved issues with them into the next relationship—or they ignore their issues and remain single.

Divorce doesn't resolve the conflict between you. You will still be sad and discouraged after the divorce is final. And if you share children, your spouse will always be a part of your life at holidays and family events.

Divorce is a family affair; it's not just between a husband and wife. Statistics prove that your children will be affected for the rest of their lives, even after they've matured and married and left home.

Divorce should be a last resort, when everything else has failed.

Divorce is emotionally devastating—for everyone.

To be honest with you, being single is not all it's cracked up to be.

It takes a huge amount of courage to stay in a troubled marriage and work things out. It will be the hardest work you've ever done. You are the only one who can decide if it's worth it to you.

Keys To Understanding

• Conflict happens.

• When people divorce, they take their unre-solved issues into the next relationship.

• Divorce is a family affair; it's not just between a husband and wife.

• Don't divorce until everything else has failed.

• You are the only person who can decide if sticking it out is worth it to you.

SIXTEEN:

What To Do When You Know It's Over

"I was born when she kissed me. I died when she left me. I lived a few weeks while she loved me."
Humphrey Bogart
In A Lonely Place. 1950

Sometimes no matter how hard you try or how many changes you make it still isn't enough. It takes two people to make a marriage and, although you can individually influence what happens, sometimes the other party simply isn't willing to cooperate. Often when a woman makes up her mind that she wants out of the relationship, there is very little you can do about it. You can plead, promise and beg and it still won't make any difference. Maybe the changes you made came too late in the relationship; maybe your wife has simply moved on without you. Maybe it just wasn't meant to be.

If you still love your wife, the rejection is very hard to take. It is a blow to your ego. You feel lost and abandoned. You don't know what you will do next. You are in a state of shock and disbelief. Your cortisol level is shooting up, and you probably can't sleep without a prescription aid. These are responses when you finally come to the conclusion that no matter what you do, your marriage is out of control. Your wife has decided that she doesn't love you anymore.

One of the most important things to remember when the situation gets this desperate is that your life isn't over. Yes, you feel rejected but you need to remember that rejection means nothing more than this particular relationship wasn't right for you at this particular point in time. It doesn't mean it won't be right later. (Two of my good friends got divorced and remarried later when they were more in tune with each other). It also doesn't mean that you won't be loved again. Just because one person may be rejecting you, it doesn't mean that the world is rejecting you. Just because one person may no longer find you attractive, it doesn't mean that others will see you the same way. You may be very attractive to others. As we have said earlier in this book, you have to take what is being said with a grain of salt. Your wife may be experiencing many different things at this time. Hormones may be one, a mid-life crisis another. These are things you don't have much control over. For a man this period is very difficult.

I think another thing that men have trouble with is change. We don't like it when we can't solve problems and we don't like change. When we can't change our situations because our wives don't want to cooperate, we invariably have to deal with change. One thing I've learned about why change is very hard for us is we overstate the value of what we leave behind and underestimate the value of what we gain with the change. Yes your present relationship may be over but that doesn't mean that there isn't an even better relationship down the road. There were reasons that your relationship ended. Maybe you learned a lot from the experience. Perhaps you will be better prepared for the next relationship from what you learned through this one. Life doesn't end because your relationship has ended. In fact, it could be just beginning.

When my wife left me, she said something that made a lot of sense. She said, "You have to start seeing the glass as half-full and not half-empty with my leaving. Now you can find that special person who will meet your needs much better than I ever did or could. If you look at it this way, you could be headed for the greatest happiness of your life."

When you've struggled for months to keep your marriage together, this isn't what you want to hear. But it makes sense. Marriages end for lots of reasons.

If you consider it the end of the world, you will not have a great attitude moving forward. If you look at it more as an opportunity to improve your life and improve yourself, you will be much more open to new and greater relationship opportunities in the future.

In reality as you end one relationship probably the last thing you want to think about is starting another one. You aren't ready yet because in many cases you haven't fully let go of your existing relationship. Even when the divorce has been finalized, many men still have hope of getting back together with their wives. Unfortunately this doesn't often happen. To really move forward and be open to the infinite possibilities the world has to offer you, you need to release your wife and move on. If you believe that you will find love again in the future, you will find it. If you tell yourself that you will never find love again, or that you don't deserve to be loved, those negative thoughts will hinder any future relationship opportunities.

The key to moving forward is to work on yourself and expect that good things will come into your life. Make yourself the best person you can be. If you are overweight, lose weight. If you don't have a job, get one. If you have personality quirks, work on them. Most importantly you need to believe that there *will* be life after your marriage has ended. You need to believe that love is still out there for you and that, yes, you can be happy again.

In her wonderful book, *Love Will Find You—9 Magnets To Bring You And Your Soulmate Together*, Kathryn Alice talks about changing your energy and becoming a magnet for love. She provides several steps for attracting your soulmate. She basically says that the only requirement for finding your soulmate is believing that true love is out there for you and having enough faith and trust in God to help you find it.

When one is going through a painful relationship breakup, one often turns to God as a last resort. When we can't understand why something is happening to us, we look for explanations from a higher power. You may consider this as a life-ending event. You may feel that there will never be anyone out there for you. You may feel abandoned and betrayed. You may be very angry with your wife. You may have even considered suicide. If you don't have someone with whom you can share your pain, major depression could set in. If you are lucky, you have your friends to talk to, but then, they have their own lives to deal with. You have professional counselors, but how do you know you have a good one?

The fact of the matter is that it doesn't cost anything to talk to God. Perhaps you cannot see the positives in the ending of your relationship. God may have something much better planned for you. So keep yourself open to love and let God do the rest. Positive expectancy is a key here.

Keys to Understanding

• *Rejection means only that this particular relationship wasn't right at this particular time.*

• *Work on yourself and expect good things to come into your life.*

• *Life doesn't end because your relationship is ending.*

• *It doesn't cost anything to talk to God, who may have something much better planned for you. Keep yourself open to love and let God do the rest.*

• *Have a sense of positive expectancy.*

Afterword:

Relationships are never easy. They take a lot of hard work and we know that most relationships aren't perfect. Long-term relationships filled with love and passion are extraordinary but they are never perfect. Those of us who are seeking perfection will always be disappointed.

Sometimes unexpected forces can enter even the most successful relationships. I have written about some of these in this book. While I truly hope that some of the information in this book will help save some marriages, I really wrote it for those good men, good husbands, good partners and good providers who will be thrust into a world neither they nor their partners understand. The good news is that as painful as the struggle to understand can become, there is (one way or another), a better day ahead. To those of you who took the time to read through this book, I hope that it has helped you to better understand this difficult and emotionally draining stage of life that is all too common. I also hope that it has provided you with some tools that you can use to survive this challenging period.

We are here at the Foundation to help you in any way we can. While this book has plenty of information to help you succeed in your journey, our website has even more resources. There is an extensive reading list on our site as well as information on various supplements discussed in the book. You will also find articles of interest as well as additional resources. Our blog will keep you current on the Foundation's activities.

Also, we enjoy nothing more than hearing from people who have been helped in some way by this book and other Foundation activities. If you would like to order additional copies for your friends or your church group, please check out the quantity prices on our website. Send us your story! It will help us fine-tune our message and help us be more effective.

You can e-mail us at **info@menonpause.org**

You can call us at **407-261-0218 or 1-888-895-2961.**

For information on having the author or one of our staff consultants speak at your event or if you would like to hear about *Where Did My Wife Go* personal coaching or our ongoing projects, including seminars and work-shops, please contact Alice Anderson at Alice@menon-pause.org

Bibliography:

Alice, Kathryn, YEAR, *Love Will Find You—9 Magnets to Bring You And Your Soulmate Together*, Da Capo Press, 2007, Cambridge, Mass.

Anton, Bill, *Neurotransmitter Deficiency Disorder*, Age, Diagnostic Laboratories, Boca Raton, Florida.

Arp, David and Claudia, 1996, *The Second Half of Marriage*, Zondervan, Grand Rapids, Michigan.

Bodmer, Judy, 1999, *When Love Dies*, Thomas Nelson, Nashville, Tennessee.

Brizendine, Louann, 2006 *The Female Brain*, Broadway Books, N.Y.,N.Y

Dayton, Tian, 2003, *The Magic of Forgiveness,* Health Communications, Inc., Deerfield Beach, Florida.

Doherty, William J., 2001, *Take Back Your Marriage,* The Guilford Press, New York/London.

Fertel, Mort, 2005, *Put Love First*, DVD.

Fertel, Mort, 2005, *Marriage Fitness*, CDs.

Fertel, Mort, 2006, *That's What I Was Going To Ask*, CDs.

Froehlich, Mary Ann, 2005, *When You're Facing the Empty Nest*, Bethany House Publishers, Minneapolis, Minnesota.

Goldstein, Andrew, Brandan, Marianne, 2004, *Reclaiming Desire*, Rodale, Inc.

Hall, Kathryn, 2004, *Reclaiming Your Sexual Self*, John Wiley & Sons, Hoboken, New Jersey.

Harris, Blase, 1989, *How To Get Your Lover Back*, Dell Publishing, New York.

Hendrix, Harville, 1988, *Getting The Love You Want*, Henry Holt & Company, LLC, New York.

Leman, Kevin, 2007, *7 Things He'll Never Tell You*, Tyndale House Publishers, Carol Stream, Illinois.

Lerner, Harriet, 1989, *The Dance of Intimacy*, Harper Collins Publishers, New York.

Lieberman, David J., 2005, *How to Change Anybody*, St. Martin's Griffin, New York.

McMahon, Susanna, *The Portable Therapist*, 1992, Dell Publishing, New York.

Markman, Howard J., Stanley, Scott M., Blumberg, Susan L., *Fighting for Your Marriage*, 2001, John Wiley & Sons, Inc., San Francisco, California.

Notarius, Clifford, Markman, Howard, Ph.D., 1993, *We Can Work It Out*, Berkley Publishing Group, New York.

Page, Susan, 1998, *How One of You Can Bring the Two of You Together*, Broadway Doubleday Dell, New York.

Page, Susan, 2006, *Why Talking Is Not Enough*, John Wiley & Sons, Inc., San Francisco, California.

Redmond, Geoffrey, 2005, *The Hormonally Vulnerable Woman*, Harper Collins Publishers, New York.

Reiss, Uzzi, 2001, *Natural Hormone Balance*, Pocket Books, New York.

Roth, Dick, *No, It's Not Hot In Here*, 1999, Ant Hill Press, Georgetown, Massachusetts.

Schlessinger, Laura, 2004, *The Proper Care & Feeding of Husbands,* Harper Collins Publishers, New York.

Schlessinger, Laura, 2004, *Woman Power*, Harper Collins Publishers, New York.

Smalley, Greg and Paul, Robert S., *The DNA of Relationships for Couples*, 2006, The Smalley Group/Tyndale House Publishers, Carol Stream, Illinois.

Vogt, Max, 2007, *You Don't Have to Change Who You Are to Have a Great Marriage,* Morgan James Publishing, Garden City, New York.

Weiner-Davis, Michele, 1992, *Divorce Busting*, Simon and Schuster Paperbacks, New York.

Weiner Davis, Michele, 2001, *The Divorce Remedy*, Simon and Schuster Paperbacks, New York.

Wright, Jonathan V., Morgenthaler, John, 1997, *Natural Hormone Replacement,* Petaluma, California.

MW01634660

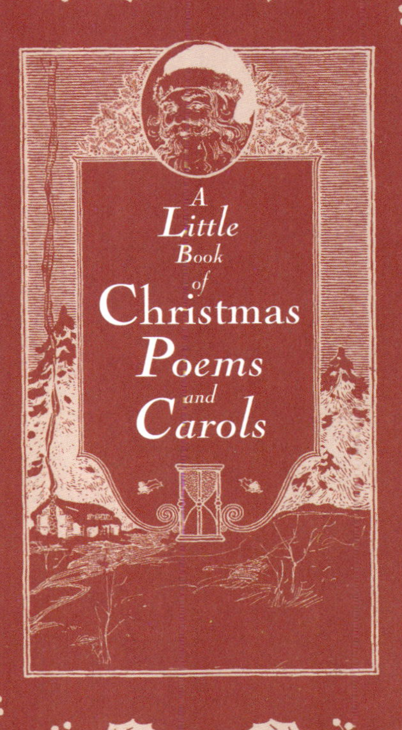
A
Little
Book
of
Christmas
Poems
and
Carols

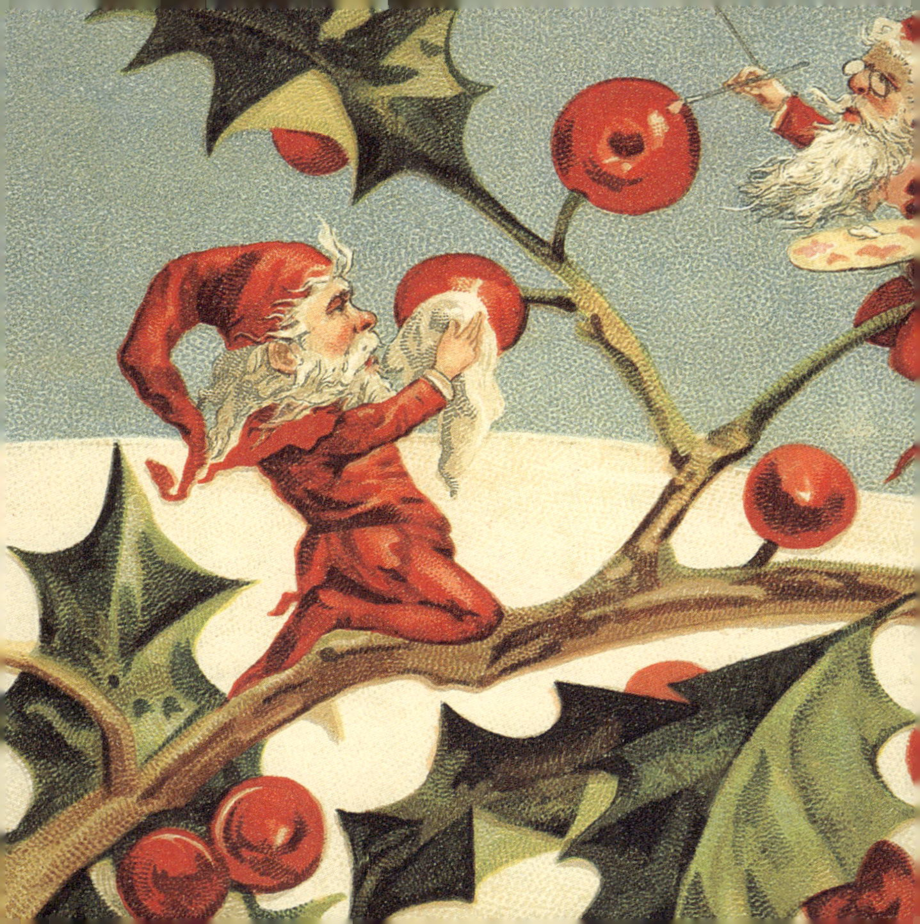

A *Little* Book of CHRISTMAS

Poems and Carols

Edited by
Lena Tabori

A Welcome Book

Andrews McMeel
Publishing

Kansas City

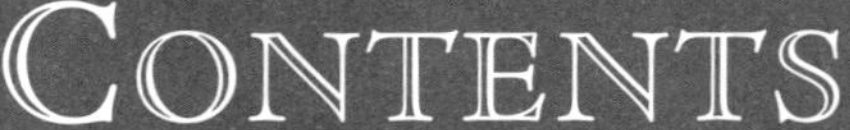CONTENTS

POEMS

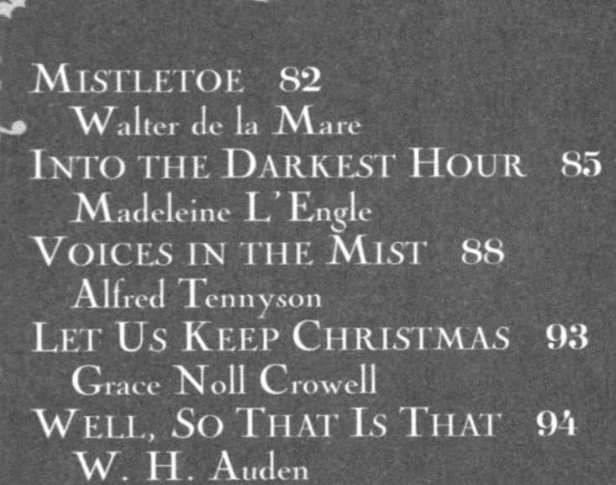

CAROLS

Christmas Eve at Sea

JOHN MASEFIELD

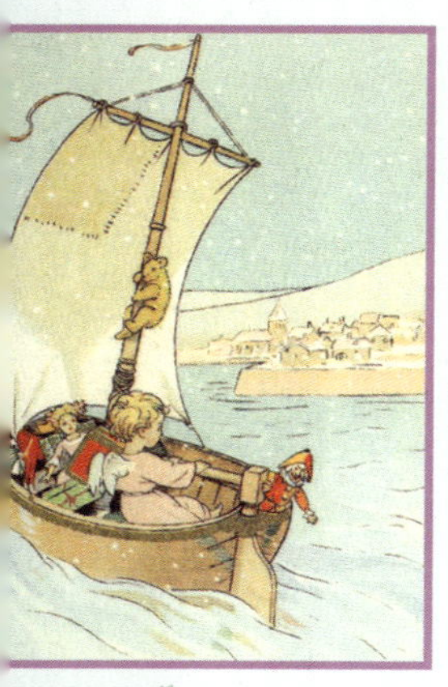

A wind is rustling "south and soft,"
  Cooing a quiet country tune,
The calm sea sighs, and far aloft
  The sails are ghostly in the moon.

Unquiet ripples lisp and purr,
  A block there pipes and chirps i' the sheave,
The wheel-ropes jar, the reef-points stir
  Faintly—and it is Christmas Eve.

The hushed sea seems to hold her breath,
  And o'er the giddy, swaying spars,
Silent and excellent as Death,
  The dim blue skies are bright with stars.

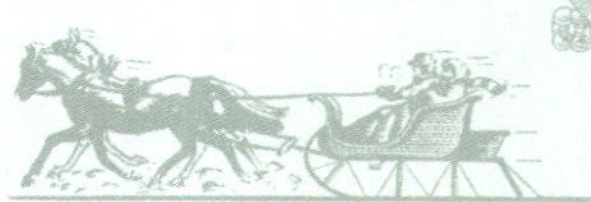

Dear God—they shone in Palestine
   Like this, and yon pale moon serene
Looked down among the lowing kine
   On Mary and the Nazarene.

The angels called from deep to deep,
   The burning heavens felt the thrill,
Startling the flocks of silly sheep
   And lonely shepherds on the hill.

To-night beneath the dripping bows,
   Where flashing bubbles burst and throng,
The bow-wash murmurs and sighs and soughs
   A message from the angels' song.

The moon goes nodding down the west,
   The drowsy helmsman strikes the bell;
Rex Judaeorum natus est,
   I charge you, brothers, sing *Nowell,*
Nowell,
Rex Judaeorum natus est

The First Noel

1. The First Noel the angels did say
   Was to certain poor shepherds in fields as they lay,
   In fields where they lay keeping their sheep,
   On a cold winter's night that was so deep.

(Chorus) Noel, Noel, Noel, Noel,
   Born is the King of Israel.

2. They looked up and saw a star
   Shining in the East beyond them far,
   And to the earth it gave great light,
   And so it continued both day and night.

(Chorus)

3. This star drew nigh to the Northwest,
   O'er Bethlehem it took its rest,
   And there it did both stop and stay,
   Right over the place where Jesus lay.

(Chorus)

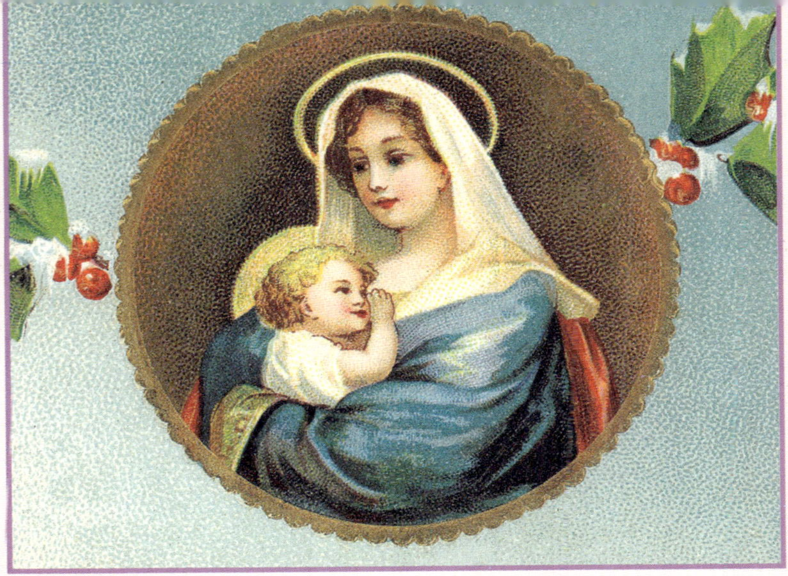

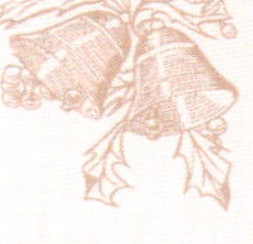

4. Then entered in those wisemen three,
   Full rev'rently upon their knee,
   And offered there in His presence,
   Their gold and myrrh and frankincense.

(Chorus)

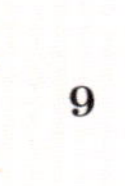
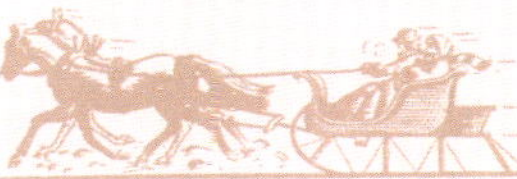

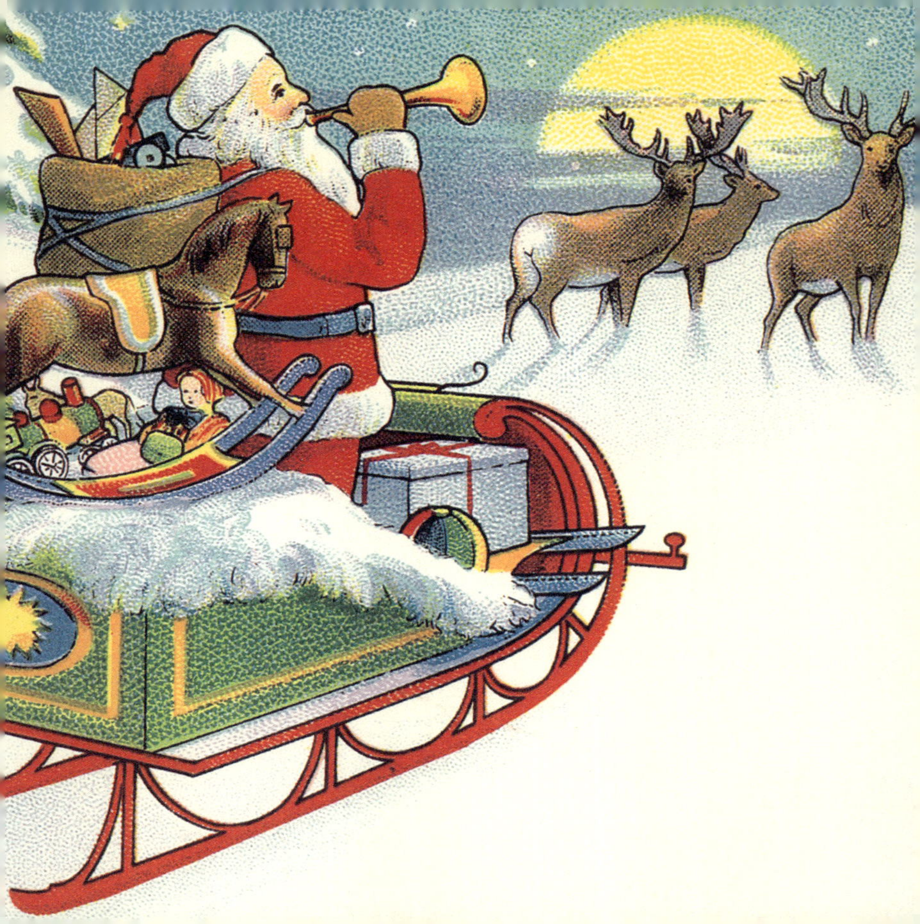

A Visit from St. Nicholas

CLEMENT CLARKE MOORE

'Twas the night before Christmas, when all through the house
Not a creature was stirring, not even a mouse.
The stockings were hung by the chimney with care,
In hopes that St. Nicholas soon would be there.
The children were nestled all snug in their beds,
While visions of sugar-plums danced in their heads;
And mamma in her kerchief, and I in my cap,
Had just settled our brains for a long winter's nap—
When out on the lawn there arose such a clatter
I sprang from my bed to see what was the matter.
Away to the window I flew like a flash,
Tore open the shutter, and threw up the sash.
The moon on the breast of the new-fallen snow
Gave a lustre of midday to objects below;
When what to my wondering eye should appear

But a miniature sleigh and eight tiny reindeer,
With a little old driver, so lively and quick,
I knew in a moment it must be St. Nick!
More rapid than eagles his coursers they came,
And he whistled and shouted and called them by name.
"Now, Dasher! now, Dancer! now, Prancer and Vixen!
On, Comet! on, Cupid! on, Donder and Blitzen!—
To the top of the porch, to the top of the wall,
Now, dash away, dash away, dash away all!"
As dry leaves that before the wild hurricane fly,
When they meet with an obstacle mount to the sky,
So, up to the housetop the coursers they flew,
With a sleigh full of toys—and St. Nicholas, too.
And then, in a twinkling, I heard on the roof
The prancing and pawing of each little hoof.
As I drew in my head and was turning around,
Down the chimney St. Nicholas came with a bound:
He was dressed all in fur from his head to his foot,
And his clothes were all tarnished with ashes and soot:
A bundle of toys he had flung on his back,
And he looked like a peddler just opening his pack.
His eyes, how they twinkled! his dimples, how merry!

His cheeks were like roses, his nose like a cherry;
His droll little mouth was drawn up like a bow,
And the beard on his chin was as white as the snow.
The stump of a pipe he held tight in his teeth,
And the smoke, it encircled his head like a wreath.
He had a broad face and a little round belly
That shook, when he laughed, like a bowl full of jelly.
He was chubby and plump—a right jolly old elf:
And I laughed when I saw him, in spite of myself;
A wink of his eye, and a twist of his head,
Soon gave me to know I had nothing to dread.
He spoke not a word, but went straight to his work,
And filled all the stockings: then turned with a jerk,
And laying his finger aside of his nose,
And giving a nod, up the chimney he rose.
He sprang to his sleigh, to his team gave a whistle,
And away they all flew like the down of a thistle.
But I heard him exclaim, ere they drove out of sight,
"Happy Christmas to all, and to all a good-night!"

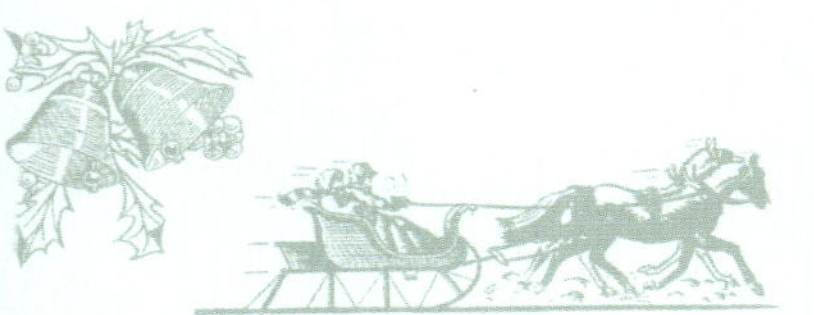

Silent Night

1. Silent night! Holy night!
all is calm, all is bright.
'Round yon virgin mother and child.
Holy infant so tender and mild,
sleep in heavenly peace,
sleep in heavenly peace.

2. Silent night! Holy night!
Shepards quake at the sight!
Glories stream from heaven afar,
Heav'nly hosts sing Alleluia,
Christ, the Saviour, is born!
Christ, the Saviour, is born!

3. Silent night! Holy night!
Son of God, love's pure light,
Radiant beams from Thy holy face,
With the dawn of redeeming grace,
Jesus, Lord, at Thy birth!
Jesus, Lord, at Thy birth!

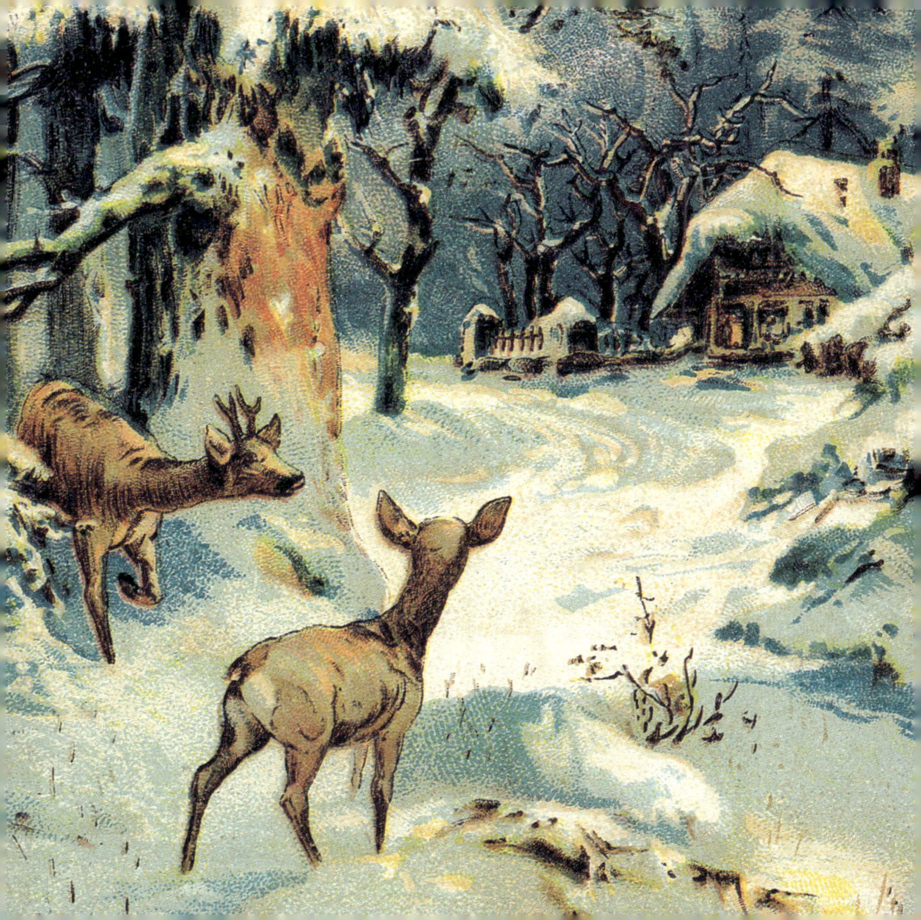

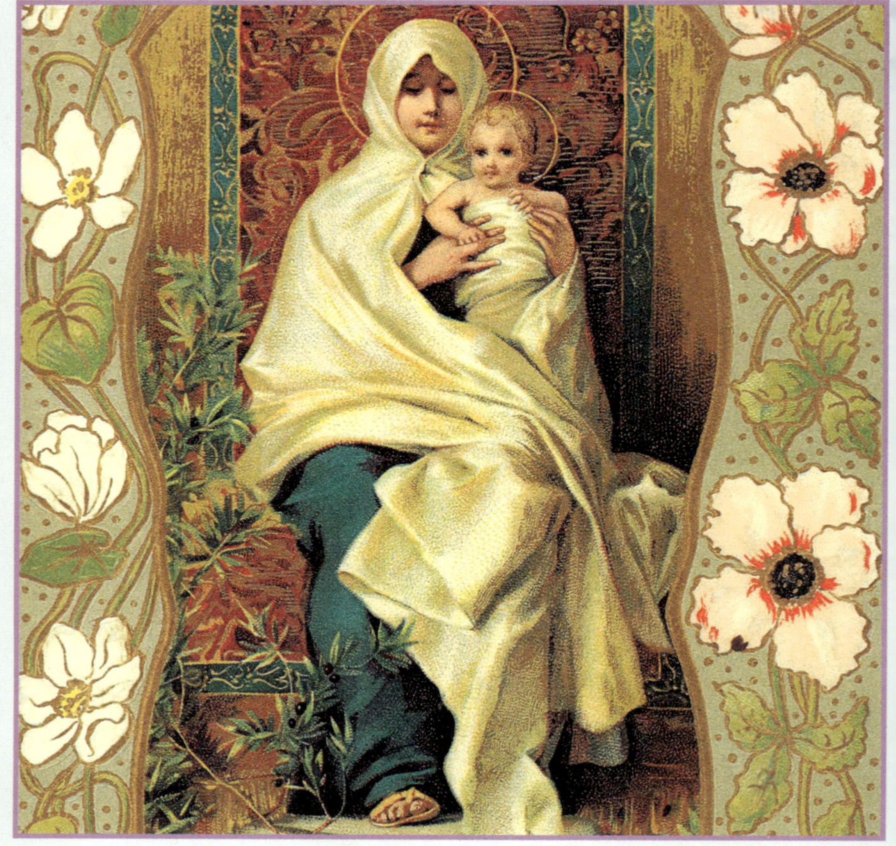

Before the Paling of the Stars

CHRISTINA G. ROSSETTI

Before the paling of the stars,
   Before the winter morn,
Before the earliest cock crow,
   Jesus Christ was born;
Born in a stable,
   Cradled in a manger,
In the world His hands had made
   Born a stranger.

Priest and king lay fast asleep
   In Jerusalem,
Young and old lay fast asleep
   In crowded Bethlehem;

Saint and Angel, ox and ass,
   Kept a watch together
Before the Christmas daybreak
   In the winter weather.

Jesus on His mother's breast
   In the stable cold,
Spotless Lamb of God was He,
   Shepherd of the fold:
Let us kneel with Mary maid,
   With Joseph bent and hoary,
With Saint and Angel, ox and ass,
   To hail the King of Glory.

O Come, All Ye Faithful

1. O Come, All Ye Faithful, Joyful and triumphant,
   O come ye, O come ye to Bethlehem.
   Come and behold Him, Born the King of Angels;

(Refrain)   O come, let us adore Him,
   O come, let us adore Him,
   O come, let us adore Him,
   Christ, the Lord.

2. Sing, choirs of angels, sing in exultation,
   O sing, all ye citizens of heav'n above!
   Glory to God, all Glory in the highest.

(Refrain)

3. Yea, Lord, we greet Thee, born this happy morning,
   Jesus, to Thee be all glory giv'n;
   Word of the Father, Now in flesh appearing.

(Refrain)

A Carol for Children

OGDEN NASH

God rest you merry, Innocents,
Let nothing you dismay,
Let nothing wound an eager heart
Upon this Christmas day.

Yours be the genial holly wreaths,
The stockings and the tree;
An aged world to you bequeaths
Its own forgotten glee.

Soon, soon enough come crueler gifts,
The anger and the tears;
Between you now there sparsely drifts
A handful yet of years.

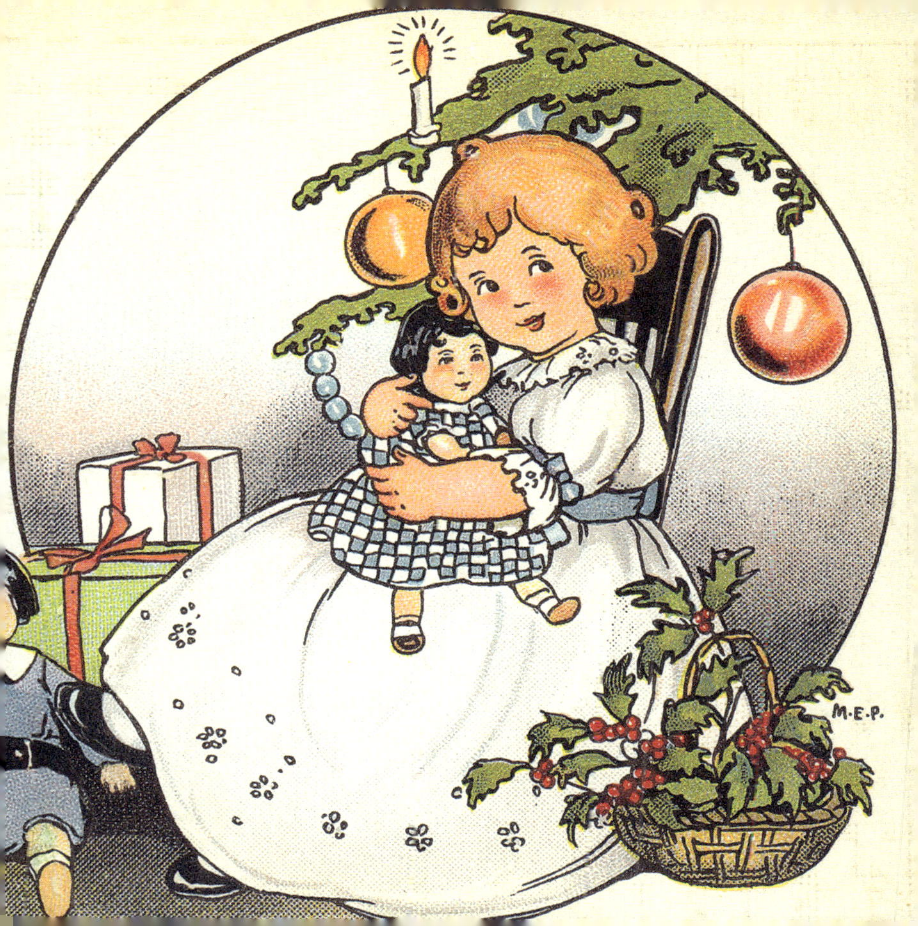

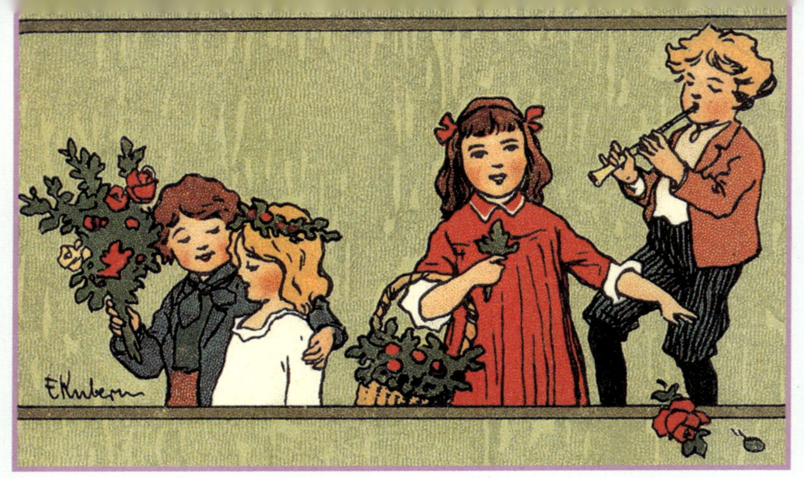

Oh, dimly, dimly glows the star
Through the electric throng;
The bidding in temple and bazaar
Drowns out the silver song.

The ancient altars smoke afresh,
The ancient idols stir;
Faint in the reek of burning flesh
Sink frankincense and myrrh.

Gaspar, Balthazar, Melchior!
Where are your offerings now?
What greetings to the Prince of War,
His darkly branded brow?

Two ultimate laws alone we know,
The ledger and the sword—
So far away, so long ago,
We lost the infant Lord.

Only the children clasp His hand;
His voice speaks low to them,
And still for them the shining band
Wings over Bethlehem.

God rest you merry, Innocents,
While Innocence endures.
A sweeter Christmas than we to ours
May you bequeath to yours.

Hark! The Herald Angels Sing

1. Hark! The Herald Angels Sing,
"Glory to the newborn King!
Peace on earth and mercy mild,
God and sinners reconciled."
Joyful all ye nations rise,
Join the triumph of the skies;
Within th' angelic host proclaim,
"Christ is born in Bethlehem."

(Refrain) Hark the Herald Angels Sing,
"Glory to the newborn King!"

2. Christ, by highest heaven adored;
Christ, the everlasting Lord;
Come, Desire of Nations, come,
Fix in us thy humble home.
Veiled in flesh the Godhead see;
Hail th' Incarnate Deity,

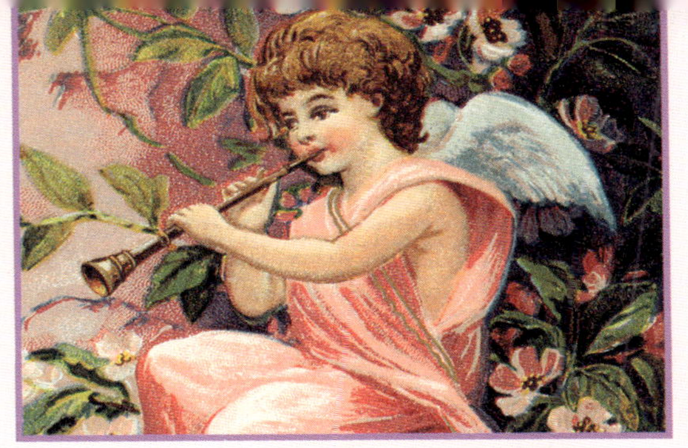

Pleased as man with man to dwell;
Jesus, our Emmanuel.

(Refrain)

3. Hail, the heave'nborn Prince of Peace!
   Hail, the Sun of Righteousness!
   Light and life to all He brings,
   Ris'n with healing in His wing;
   Mild He lays His glory by,
   Born that man no more may die,
   Born to raise the sons of earth,
   Born to give them second birth;

   (Refrain)

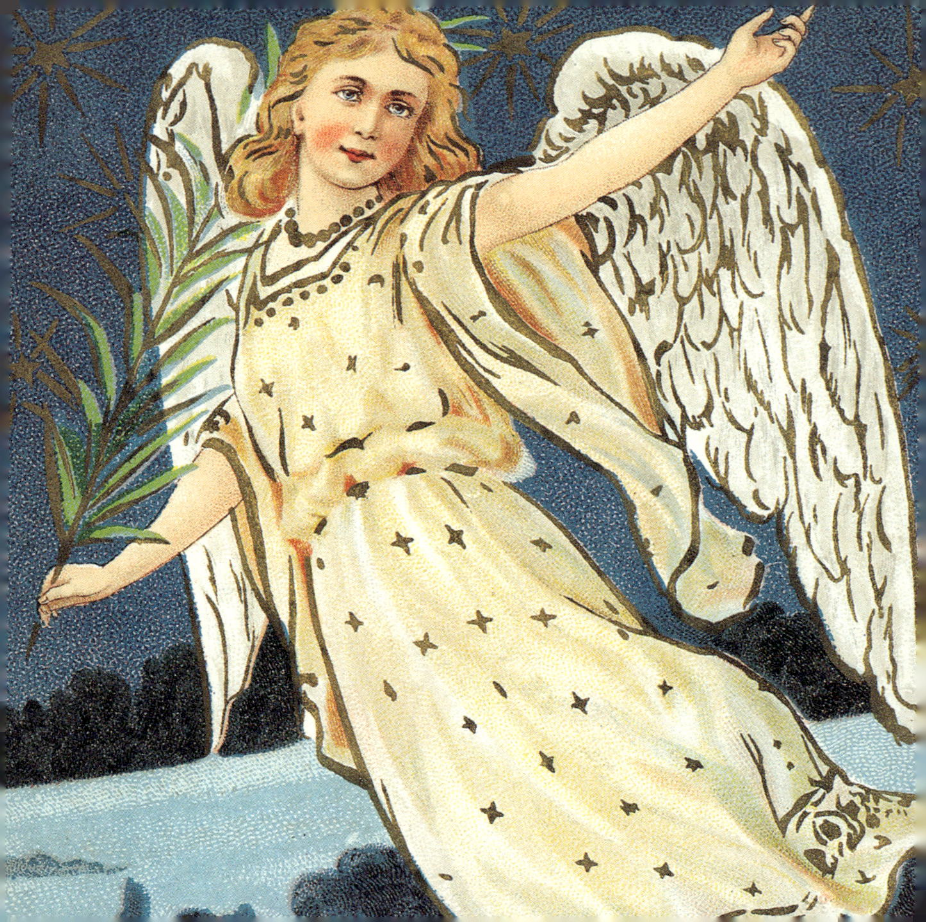

Long, Long Ago

KATHERINE PARKER

Winds through the olive trees
Softly did blow,
Round little Bethlehem
Long, long ago.

Sheep on the hillside lay
Whiter than snow;
Shepherds were watching them
Long, long ago.

Then from the happy sky
Angels bent low,
Singing their songs of joy
Long, long ago.

For in a manger bed,
Cradled we know,
Christ came to Bethlehem
Long, long ago.

We Three Kings of Orient Are

1. We Three Kings of Orient are,
Bearing gifts we traverse afar,
Field and fountain, Moor and mountain,
Following yonder star.

(Refrain) O, star of wander, star of night,
Star of royal beauty bright,
Westward leading, still proceeding,
Guide us to thy perfect light.

2. Born a King on Bethlehem plain,
Gold I bring to crown Him again,
King forever, Ceasing never
Over us all to reign.

(Refrain)

3. Frankincense to offer have I,
   Incense owns a Deity night:
   Prayer and praising, All men raising,
   Worship Him, God on high.

   (Refrain)

4. Myrrh is mine; its bitter perfume
   Breathes a life of gathering gloom;
   Sorrowing, sighing, Bleeding, dying,
   Sealed in the stone cold tomb.

   (Refrain)

5. Glorious now behold Him arise,
   King and God, and sacrifice;
   Heaven sings Alleluia:
   Alleluia the earth replies.

   (Refrain)

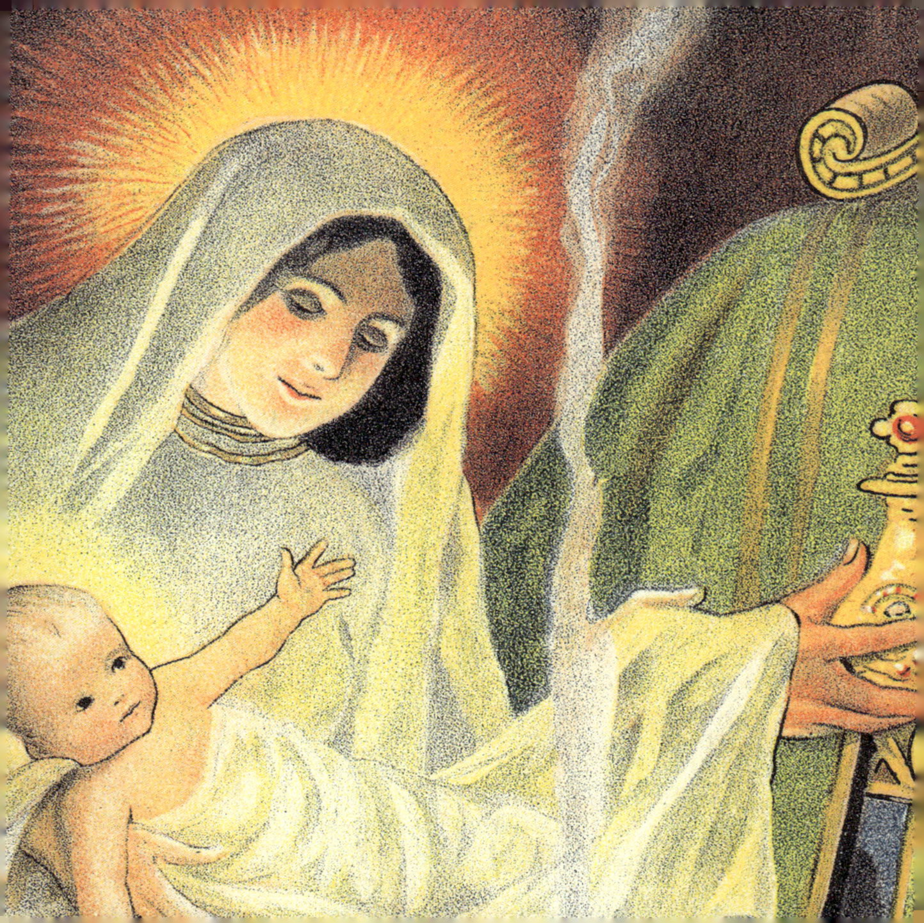

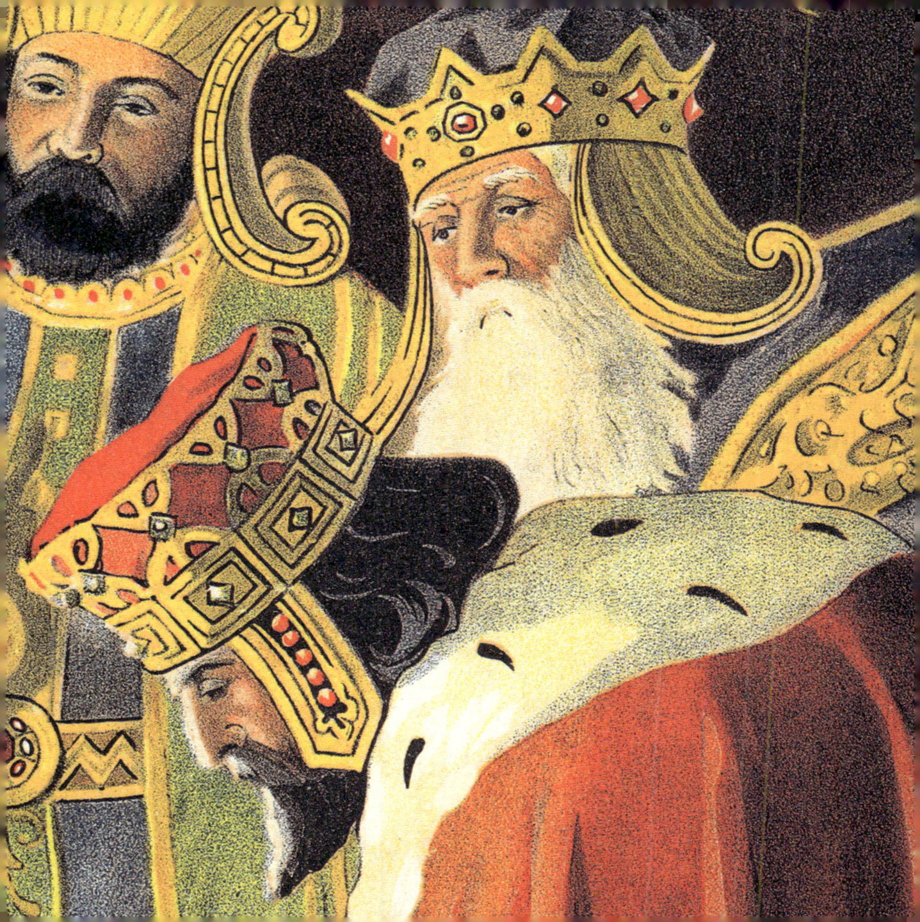

The Bells

EDGAR ALLAN POE

Hear the sledges with the bells—
    Silver bells!
What a world of merriment their melody
    foretells!
How they tinkle, tinkle, tinkle,
  In the icy air of night!
While the stars, that oversprinkle
All the heavens, seem to twinkle
  With a crystalline delight
Keeping time, time, time,
  In a sort of Runic rhyme.
To the tintinnabulation that so
    musically wells
From the bells, bells, bells, bells,
    Bells, bells, bells—
From the jingling and the tinkling of
    the bells.

The Holly and the Ivy

(Traditional English Carol)

1. The holly and the ivy,
   When they are both full grown,
   Of all the trees that are in the wood,
   The holly bears the crown.

(Refrain) The rising of the sun
   And the running of the deer,
   The playing of the merry organ,
   Sweet singing in the choir.

2. The holly bears a blossom
   As white as the lily flow'r,
   And Mary bore sweet Jesus Christ,
   To be our sweet Savior.

(Refrain)

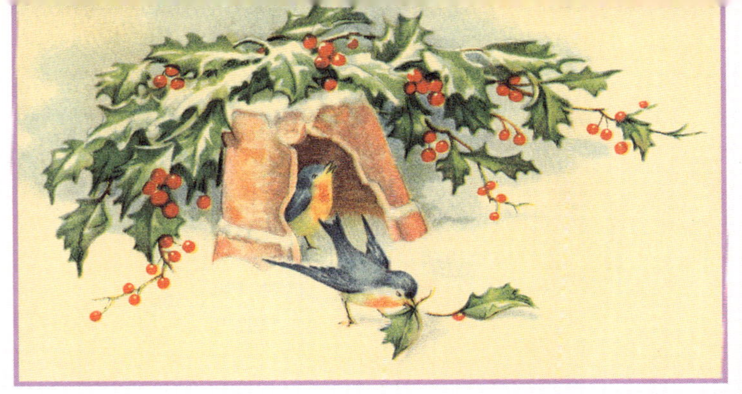

3. The holly bears a berry
   As red as any blood,
   And Mary bore sweet Jesus Christ
   To do poor sinners good.

   (Refrain)

4. The holly bears a prickle,
   As sharp as any thorn,
   And Mary bore sweet Jesus Christ
   On Christmas day in the morn.

   (Refrain)

5. The holly bears a bark,
   As bitter as any gall,
   And Mary bore sweet Jesus Christ
   For to redeem us all.

   (Refrain)

6. The holly and the ivy,
   When they are both full grown,
   Of all the trees that are in the wood,
   The holly bears the crown.

   (Refrain)

Carol of the Field Mice

from *The Wind in the Willows*
KENNETH GRAHAME

Villagers all, this frosty tide,
Let your doors swing open wide,
Though wind may follow, and snow beside,
Yet draw us in by your fire to bide;
　　Joy shall be yours in the morning!

Here we stand in the cold and the sleet,
Blowing fingers and stamping feet,
Come from far away you to greet—
you by the fire and we in the street—
　　Bidding you joy in the morning!

For ere one half of the night was gone,
Sudden a star has led us on,

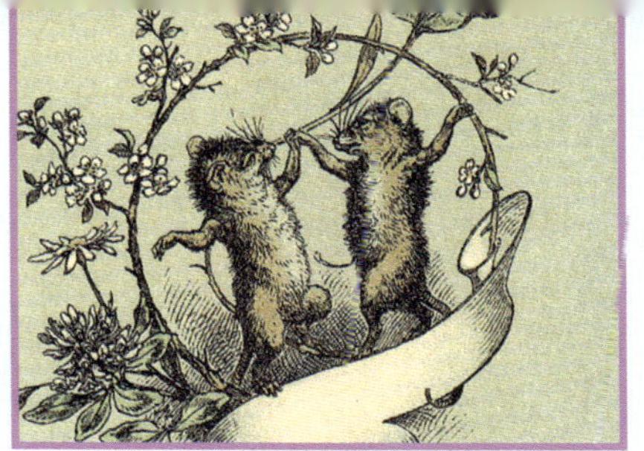

Raining bliss and benison—
Bliss tomorrow and more anon,
  Joy for every morning!

Goodman Joseph toiled through the snow—
Saw the star o'er a stable low;
Mary she might not further go—
Welcome thatch, and litter below!
  Joy was hers in the morning!

And then they heard the angels tell
"Who were the first to cry Nowell?
Animals all, as it befell,
In the stable where they did dwell!
  Joy shall be theirs in the morning!"

Jingle Bells

1. Dashing through the snow,
In a one horse open sleigh;
O'er the fields we go,
Laughing all the way.
Bells on bobtail ring,
Making spirits bright,
What fun it is to ride and sing
A sleighing song tonight.

(Chorus) Oh! Jingle Bells, Jingle Bells!
Jingle all the way!
Oh, what fun it is to ride
In a one horse open sleigh.

2. Day or two ago
I thought I'd take a ride,
Soon Miss Fanny Bright
Was seated at my side.

The horse was lean and lank,
Misfortune seem'd his lot,
He got into a drifted bank,
And we, we got upsot!

(Chorus)

3. Now the ground is white,
Go it while you're young!
Take the girls tonight,
And sing this sleighing song.
Just get a bobtail'd bay,
Twoforty for his speed,
Then hitch him to an open sleigh
And crack! You'll take the lead.

(Chorus)

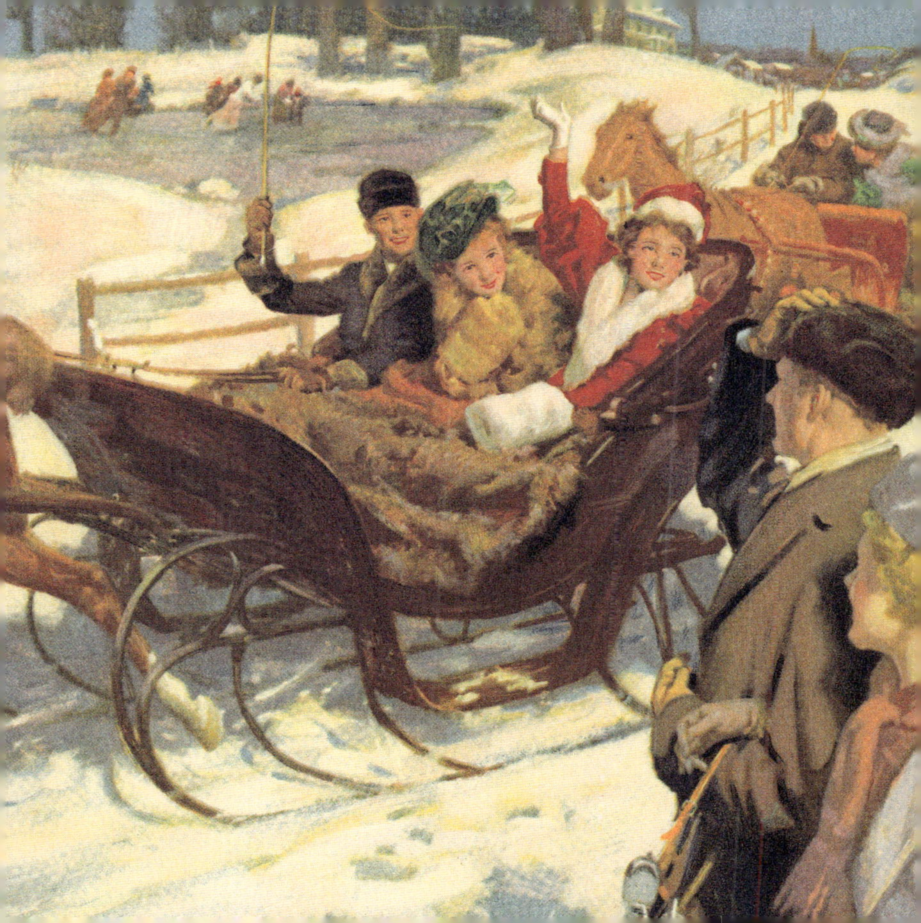

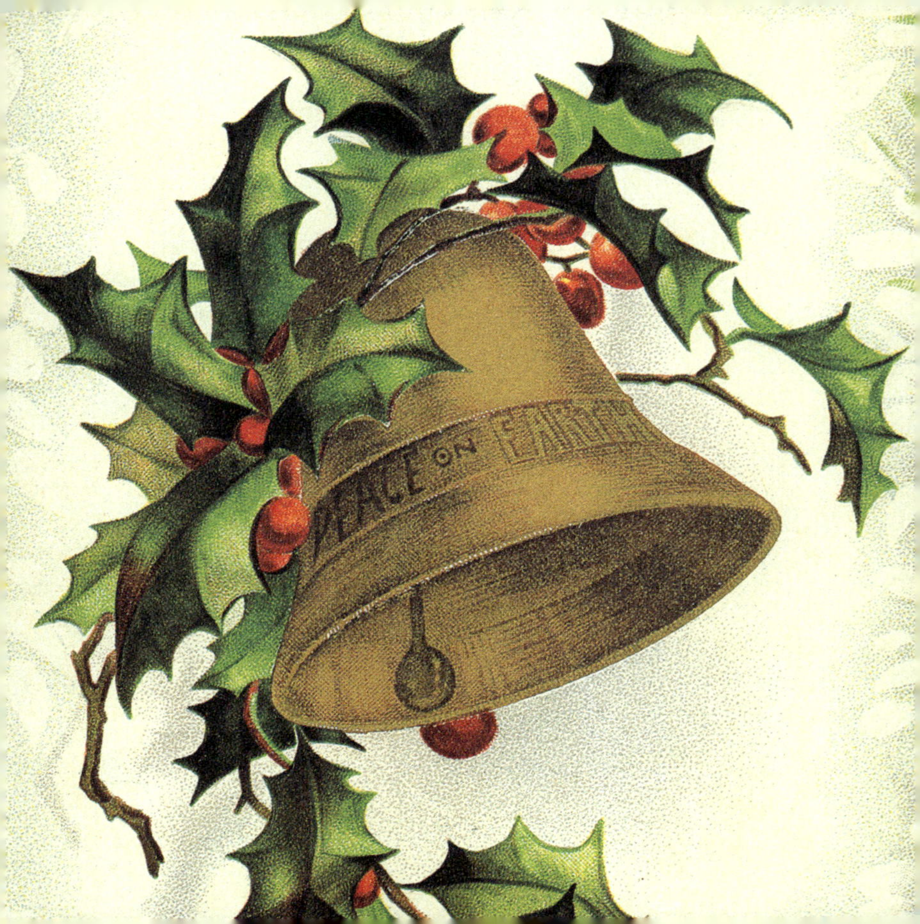
PEACE ON EARTH

Christmas Bells

HENRY WADSWORTH LONGFELLOW

I heard the bells on Christmas Day
Their old, familiar carols play,
And wild and sweet
The words repeat
Of peace on earth, good-will to men!

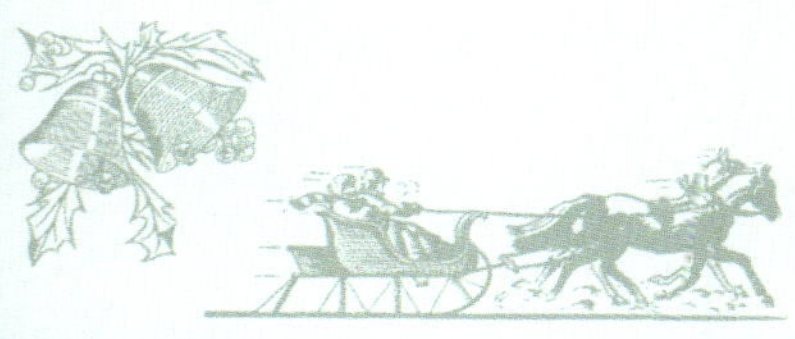

God Rest You Merry, Gentlemen

1. God Rest You Merry, Gentlemen,
let nothing you dismay,
Remember Christ our Savior
Was born on Christmas day,
To save us all from Satan's pow'r,
When we were gone astray.

(Refrain) O, tidings of comfort and joy,
Comfort and joy,
O, tidings of comfort and joy.

2. "Fear not, then," said the angel,
"Let nothing you affright,
This day is born a Savior
Of a pure Virgin bright,
To free all those who trust in Him
From Satan's power and might."

(Refrain)

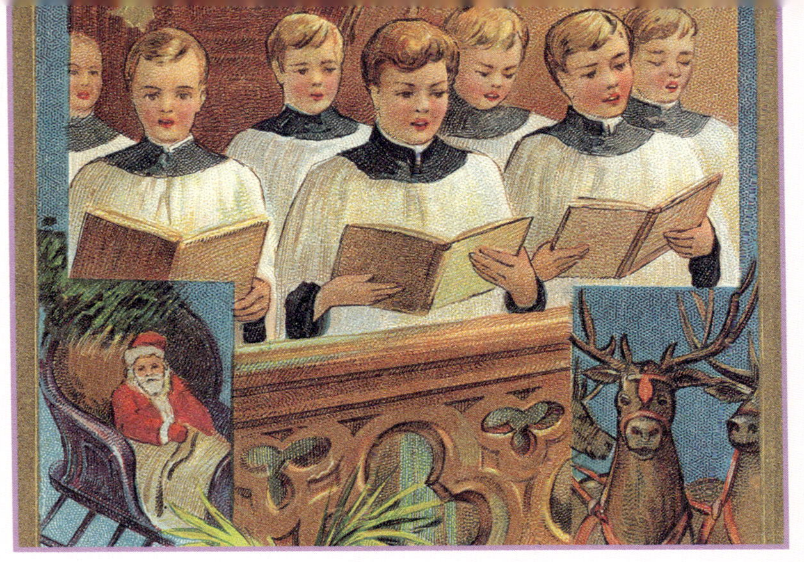

3. Now to the Lord sing praises,
All you within this place,
And with true love and brotherhood
Each other now embrace;
This holy tide of Christmas
All others doth deface.

(Refrain)

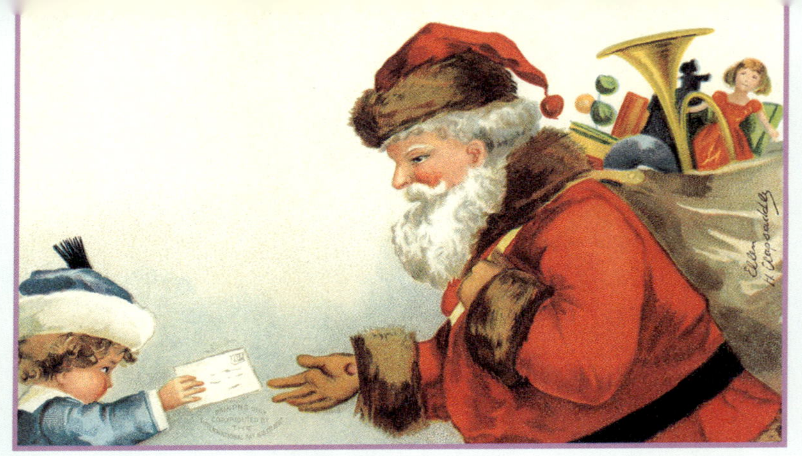

A Friend's Greeting

EDGAR A. GUEST

I'd like to be the sort of friend that you have been to me;
I'd like to be the help that you've been always glad to be;
I'd like to mean as much to you each minute of the day
As you have meant, old friend of mine, to me along the way.

I'd like to do the big things and the splendid things for you,
To brush the gray from out your skies and leave them only
   blue;
I'd like to say the kindly things that I so oft have heard,
And feel that I could rouse your soul the way that
   mine you've stirred.

I'd like to give you back the joy that you have given me,
Yet that were wishing you a need I hope will never be;
I'd like to make you feel as rich as I, who travel on
Undaunted in the darkest hours with you to lean upon.

I'm wishing at this Christmas time that I could but repay
A portion of the gladness that you've strewn along my way;
And could I have one wish this year, this only would it be:
I'd like to be the sort of friend that you have been to me.

Deck the Halls

1. Deck the Halls with boughs of holly, Fa la la la la la la la la.
'Tis the season to be jolly, Fa la la la la la la la la.
Don we now our gay apparel, Fa la la la la la la la la.
Troll the ancient Yuletide carol, Fa la la la la la la la la.

2. See the blazing Yule before us, Fa la la la la la la la la.
Strike the harp and join the chorus, Fa la la la la la la la la.
Follow me in merry measure, Fa la la la la la la la la.
While I tell of Yuletide treasure, Fa la la la la la la la la.

3. Fast away the old year passes, Fa la la la la la la la la.
Hail the new, ye lads and lasses, Fa la la la la la la la la.
Sing we joyous all together, Fa la la la la la la la la.
Heedless of the wind and weather, Fa la la la la la la la la.

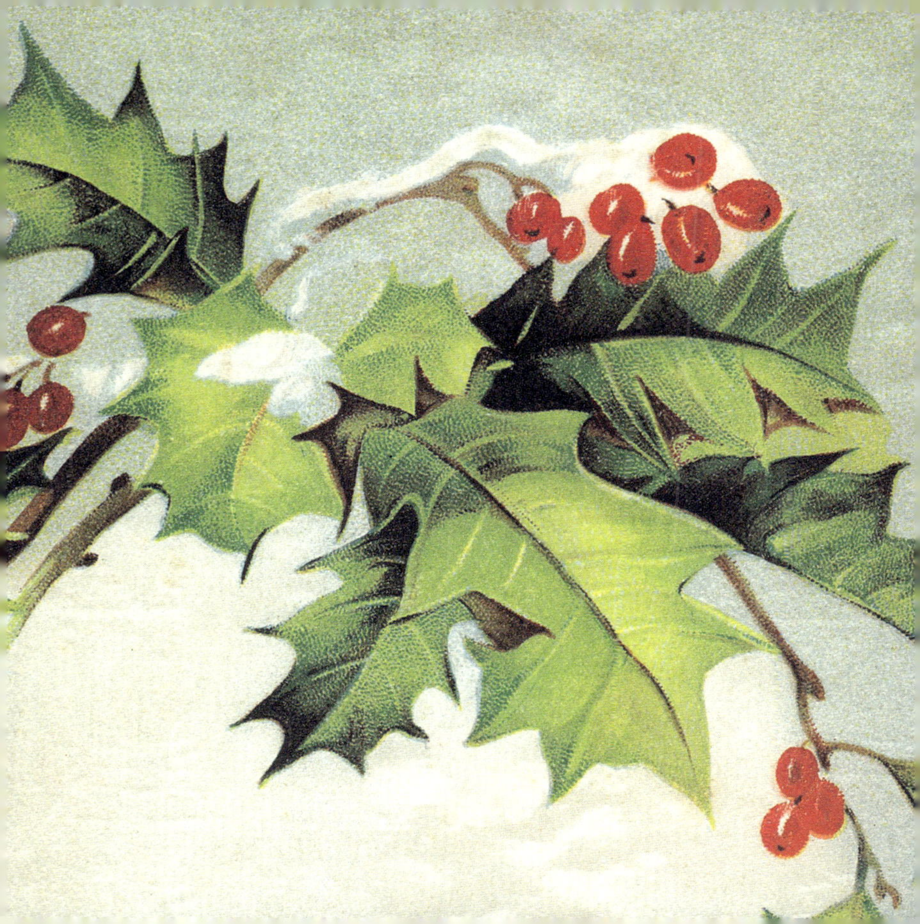

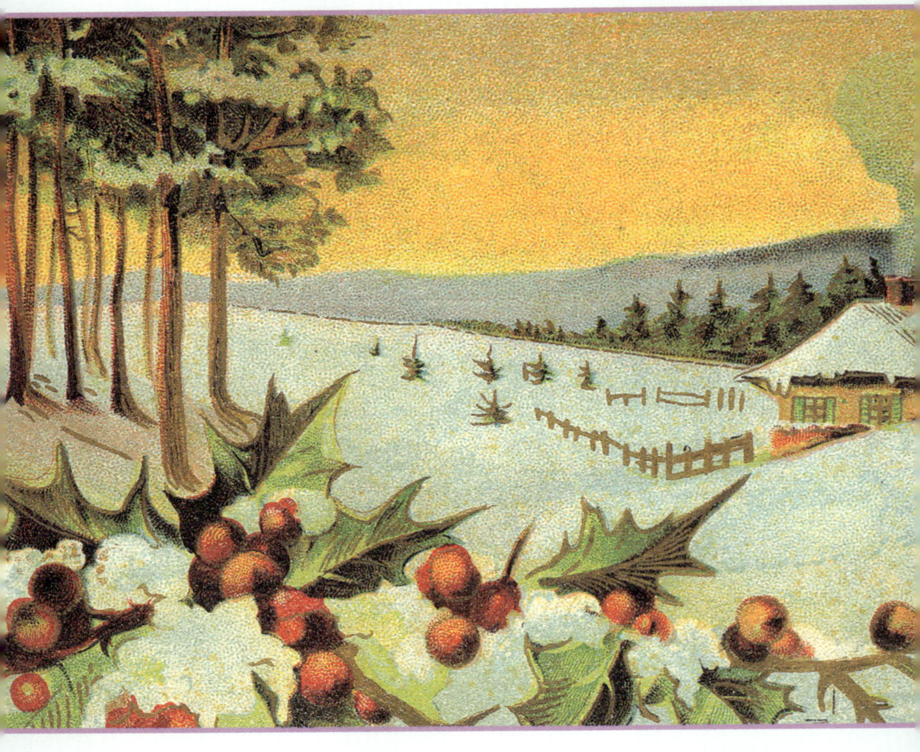

Old Irish Carol

God bless the master of this house,
　　Likewise the mistress too.
May their barns be filled with wheat
　　　　and corn,
And their hearts be always true.

A merry Christmas is our wish
　　Where'er we do appear,
To you a well-filled purse, a well-filled
　　　　dish.
And a happy bright New Year!

I Saw Three Ships

As I sat on a stormy bank,
On Christmas Day in the morning,

I spied three ships come sailing by,
On Christmas Day in the morning.

And who should be with those three ships
But Joseph and his fair lady!

One did whistle, and she did sing,
On Christmas Day in the morning,

And all the bells on earth did ring,
On Christmas Day in the morning.

For joy that our Savior He was born
On Christmas Day in the morning.

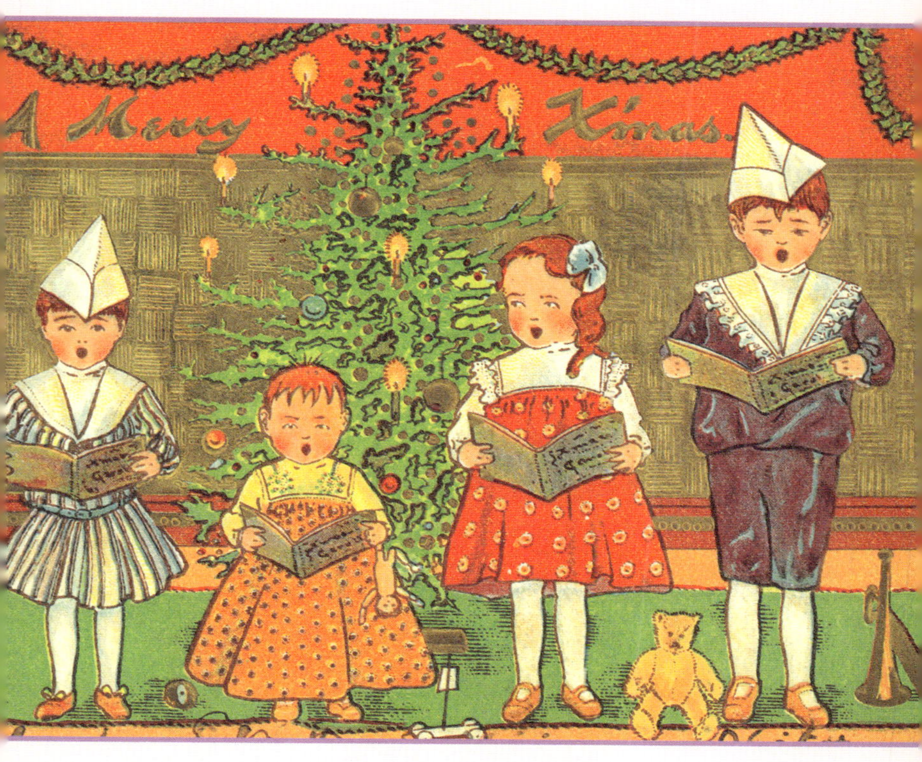

A Merry
X'mas.

The Mahogany Tree

WILLIAM MAKEPEACE THACKERAY

Christmas is here:
Winds whistle shrill,
Icy and chill,
Little care we:
Little we fear
Weather without,
Sheltered about
The Mahogany Tree.

Once on the boughs
Birds of rare plume
Sang, in its bloom;
Night-birds are we:
Here we carouse,
Singing like them,

Perched round the stem
Of the jolly old tree.

Here let us sport,
Boys, as we sit;
Laughter and wit
Flashing so free.
Life is but short—
When we are gone,
Let them sing on,
Round the old tree.
Evenings we knew,
Happy as this;
Faces we miss,
Pleasant to see.

Kind hearts and true,
Gentle and just,
Peace to your dust!
We sing round the tree.

Care, like a dun,
Lurks at the gate:
Let the dog wait;
Happy we'll be!
Drink, every one;
Pile up the coals,
Fill the red bowls,
Round the old tree!
Drain we the cup.—
Friend, art afraid?
Spirits are laid
In the Red Sea.
Mantle it up;
Empty it yet;
Let us forget,
Round the old tree.

Sorrows, begone!
Life and its ills,
Duns and their bills,
Bid we to flee.
Come with the dawn,
Blue-devil sprite,
Leave us to-night,
Round the old tree.

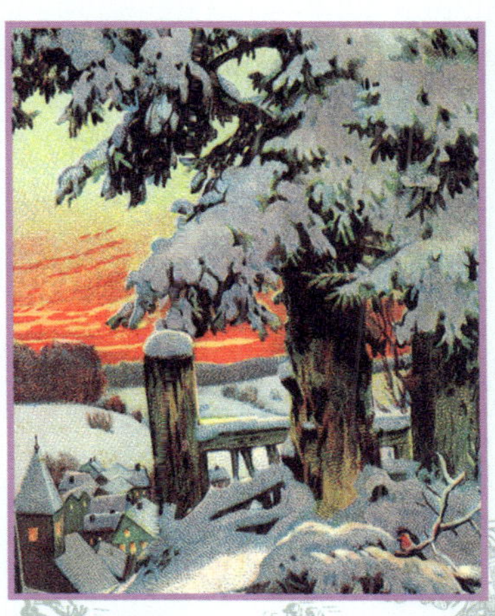

What Child Is This?

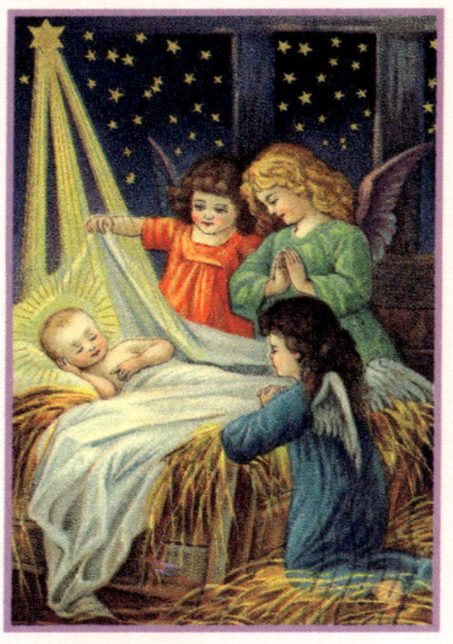

1. What Child is this, who laid to rest
   On Mary's lap, is sleeping?
   Whom angels greet with anthems sweet,
   While shepherds watch are keeping?

(Refrain) This, this is Christ the King,
Whom shepherds guard and angels sing:
Haste, haste to bring Him land,
The Babe, the Son of Mary.

2. Why lies He in such mean estate,
Where ox and ass are feeding?
Good Christians fear: for sinners here
The silent Word is pleading.

(Refrain)

3. So bring him incense, gold, and myrrh,
Come peasant, king to own Him:
The King of Kings salvation brings:
Let loving hearts enthrone Him!

(Refrain)

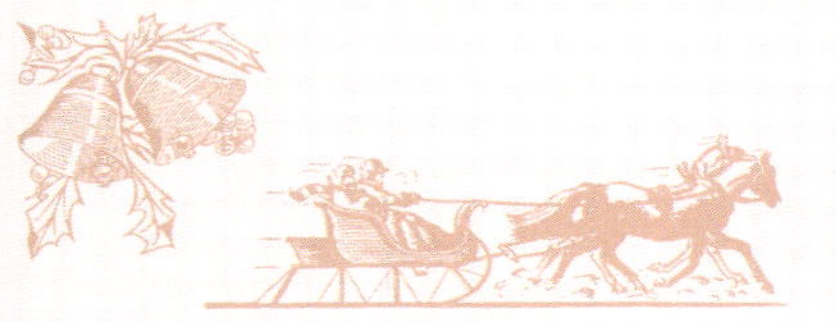

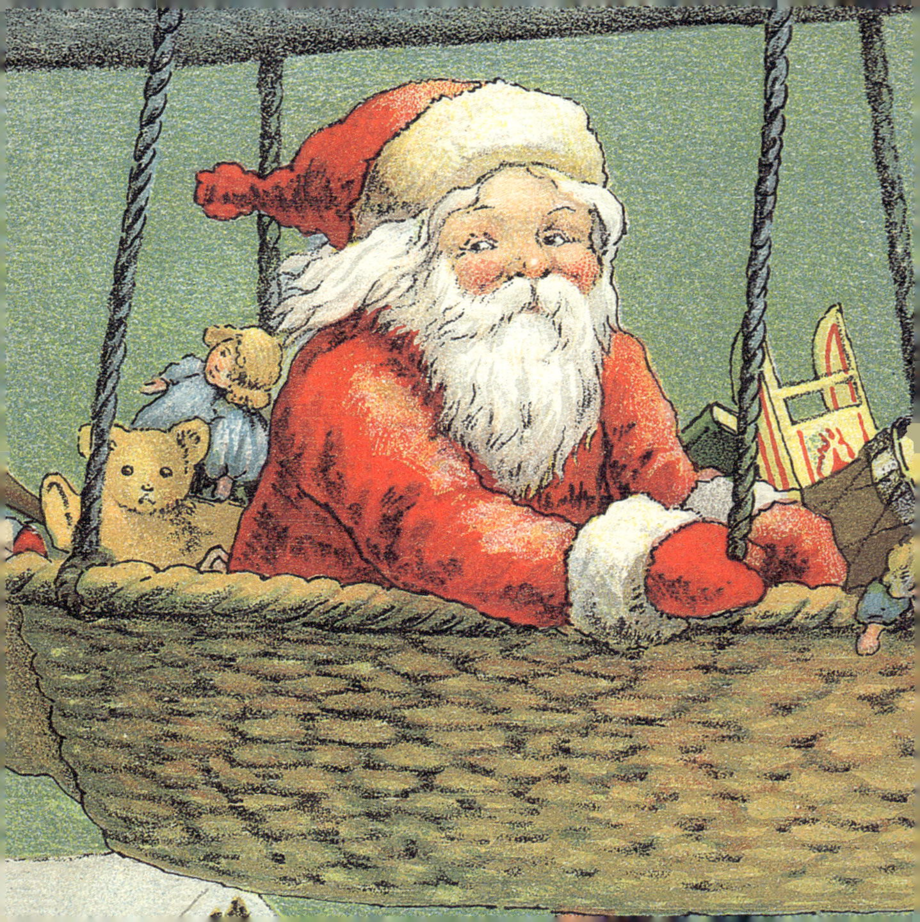

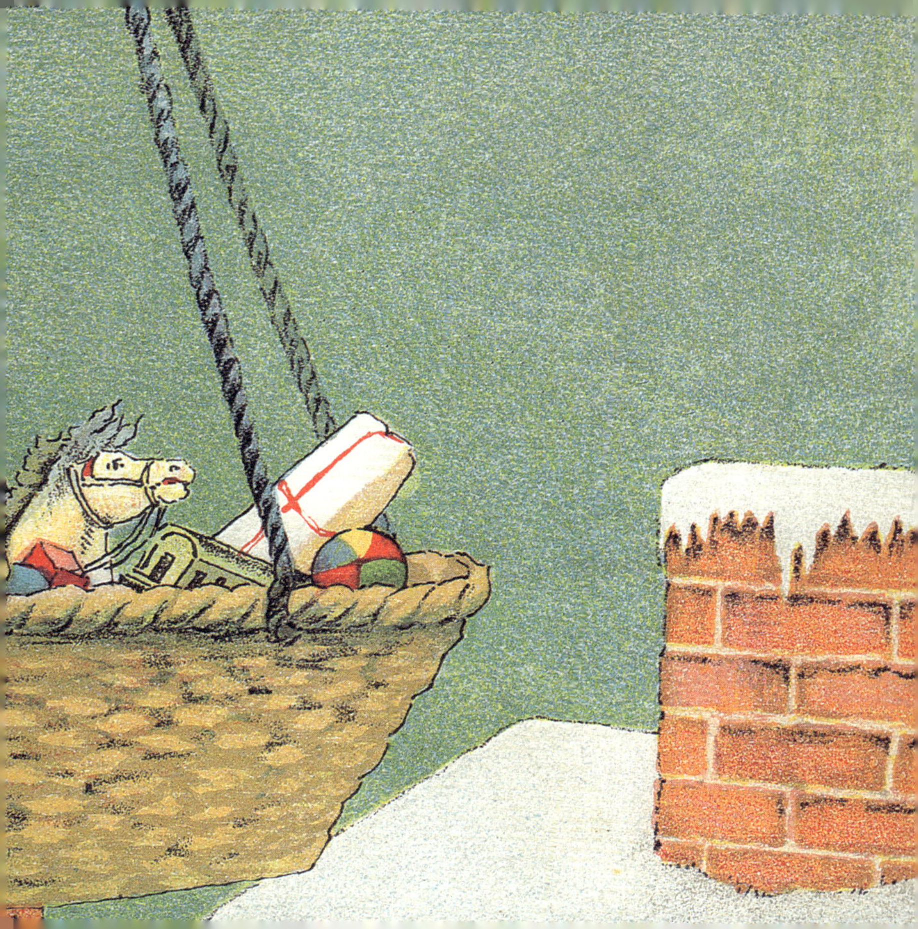

O Little Town of Bethlehem

1. O Little Town of Bethlehem,
   How still we see thee lie;
   Above thy deep and dreamless sleep
   The silent stars go by;
   Yet in thy dark streets shineth
   The everlasting light;
   The hopes and fears of all the years
   Are met in thee tonight.

2. For Christ is born of Mary,
   And gathered all above,
   While mortals sleep, the angels keep
   Their watch of wond'ring love.
   O morning stars, together
   Proclaim the holy birth!
   And praises sing to God the King,
   And peace to men on earth!

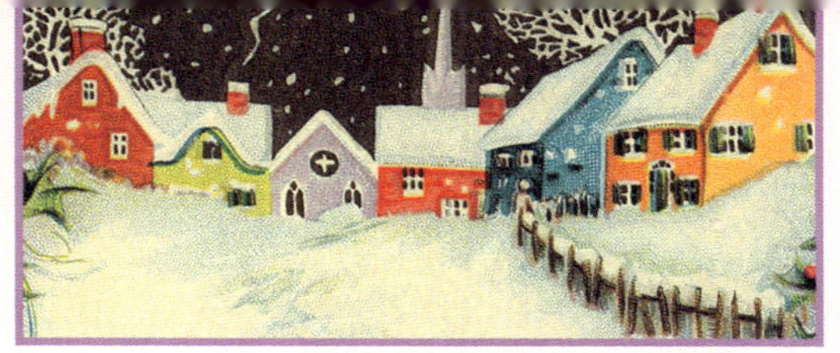

3. How silently, how silently,
   The wondrous gift is giv'n!
   So God imparts to human hearts
   The blessing of his heav'n.
   No ear may hear His coming,
   But in this world of sin,
   Where meek souls will receive Him still,
   The dear Christ enters in.

4. O Holy child of Bethlehem!
   Descent to us, we pray;
   Cast out our sin, and enter in;
   Be born in us today.
   We hear the Christmas angels
   The great glad tidings tell;
   O come to us abide with us,
   Our Lord Emmanuel.

Ring Out Wild Bells

ALFRED TENNYSON

Ring out wild bells to the wild sky,
    The flying cloud, the frosty light;
    The year is dying in the night;
Ring out, wild bells, and let him die.

Ring out the old, ring in the new,
    Ring, happy bells, across the snow;
    The year is going, let him go;
Ring out the false, ring in the true,
    Ring out the grief that saps the
        wind,
    For those that here we see no more;
    Ring out the feud of rich and poor,
Ring in redress to all mankind.

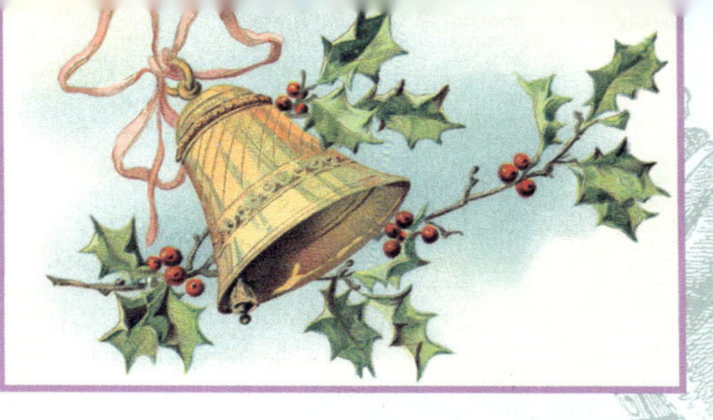

Ring out the want, the care, the sin,
  The faithless coldness of the times;
  Ring out, ring out my mournful
      rhymes,
But ring the fuller minstrel in.

Ring out old shapes of foul disease,
  Ring out the narrowing lust of gold;
  Ring out the thousand wars of old,
Ring in the thousand years of peace.

Ring in the valiant man and free,
  The larger heart, the kindlier hand;
  Ring out the darkness of the land,
Ring in the Christ that is to be.

Angels We Have Heard on High

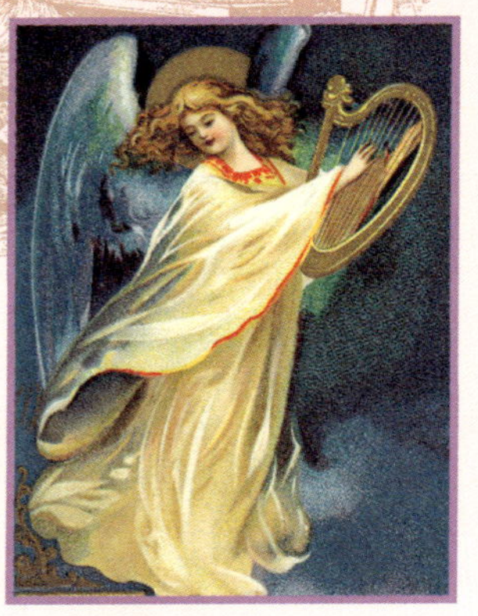

1. Angels We Heave Heard on High,
Sweetly singing o'er the plain,
And the mountains in reply,
Echoing their joyous strain.

(Refrain)   *Gloria in excelsis Deo,*
Gloria in excelsis Deo!

2. *Shepherds, why this jubilee?*
Why your joyful strains prolong?
What the gladsome tidings be
Which inspire your heav'nly song?

(Refrain)

3. *Come to Bethlehem and see*
Him whose birth the angels sing;
Come adore on bended knee
Christ, the Lord, the new-born King.

(Refrain)

4. *See Him in a manger laid,*
Whom the choir of angels praise;
Holy Spirit, lend thine aid,
While our hearts in love we raise.

(Refrain)

Christmas Greeting from a Fairy to a Child

LEWIS CARROLL

Lady, dear, if Fairies may
  For a moment lay aside
Cunning tricks and elfish play,
  'Tis at happy Christmas-tide.

We have heard the children say—
  Gentle children, whom we love—
Long ago on Christmas Day,
  Came a message from above.

Still, as Christmas-tide comes round,
  They remember it again—
Echo still the joyful sound,
  "Peace on earth, good-will to men!"

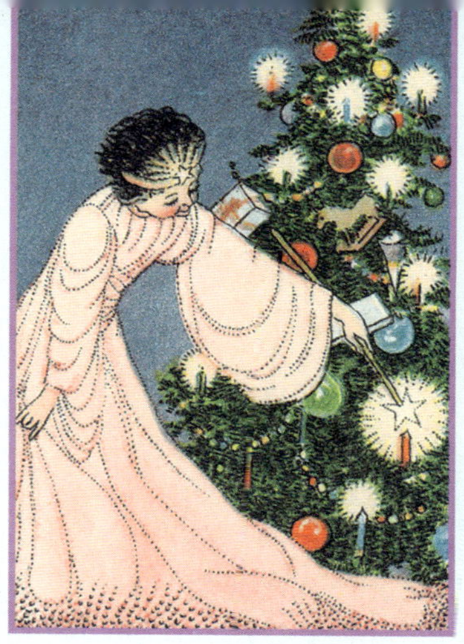

Yet the hearts must childlike be
    Where such heavenly guests abide;
Unto children, in their glee,
    All the year is Christmas-tide!

Thus, forgetting tricks and play
    For a moment, Lady dear,
We would wish you, if we may,
    Merry Christmas, glad New Year!

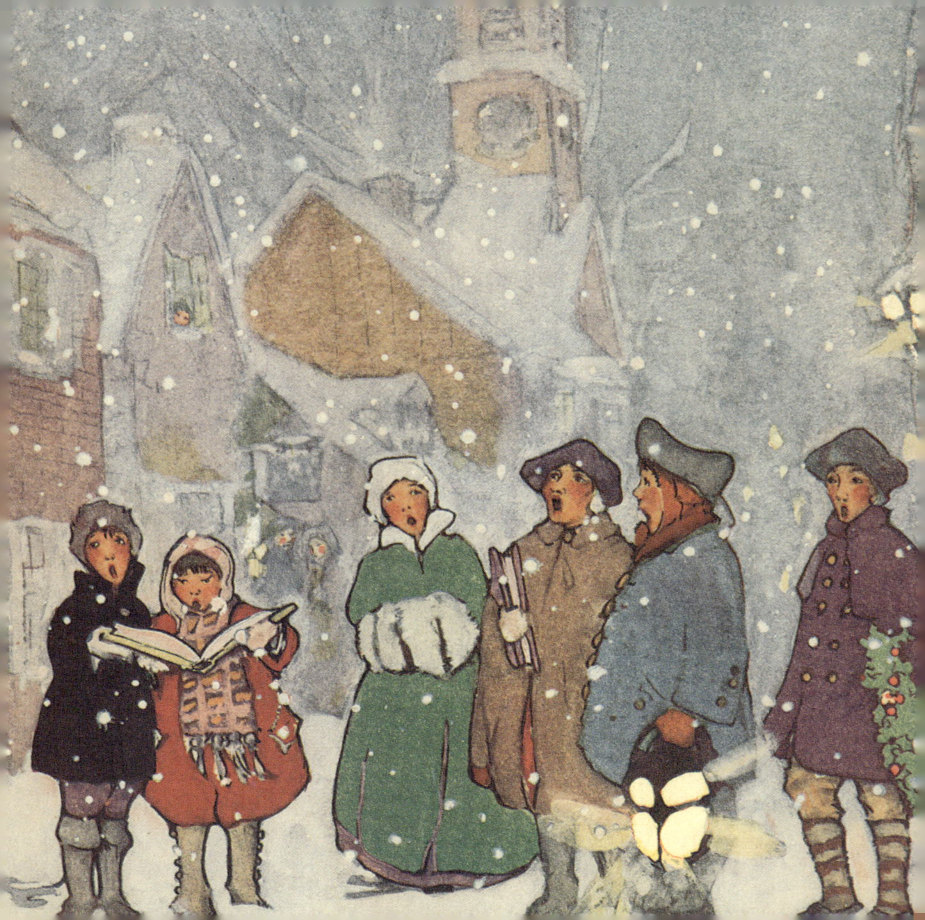

Go Tell It on the Mountain

1. When I was a seeker
   I sought both night and day,
   I asked the Lord to help me,
   And he showed me the way.

2. Go tell it on the mountain,
   Over the hills and everywhere,
   Go tell it on the mountain,
   Our Jesus Christ is born.

3. He made me a watchman
   Upon a city wall,
   And if I am a Christian,
   I am the least of all.

4. Go tell it on the mountain,
   Over the hills and everywhere,
   Go tell it on the mountain,
   Our Jesus Christ is born.

Christmas Trees: A Christmas Circular Letter

ROBERT FROST

The city had withdrawn into itself
And left at last the country to the country;
When between whirls of snow not come to lie
And whirls of foliage not yet laid, there drove
A stranger to our yard, who looked the city,
Yet did in country fashion in that there
He sat and waited till he drew us out,
A-buttoning coats, to ask him who he was.
He proved to be the city come again
To look for something it had left behind
And could not do without and keep its Christmas.
He asked if I would sell my Christmas trees;
My woods—the young fir balsams like a place

Where houses all are churches and have spires.
I hadn't thought of them as Christmas trees.
I doubt if I was tempted for a moment
To sell them off their feet to go in cars
And leave the slope behind the house all bare,
Where the sun shines now no warmer than the moon.
I'd hate to have them know it if I was.
Yet more I'd hate to hold my trees, except
As others hold theirs or refuse for them,
Beyond the time of profitable growth—

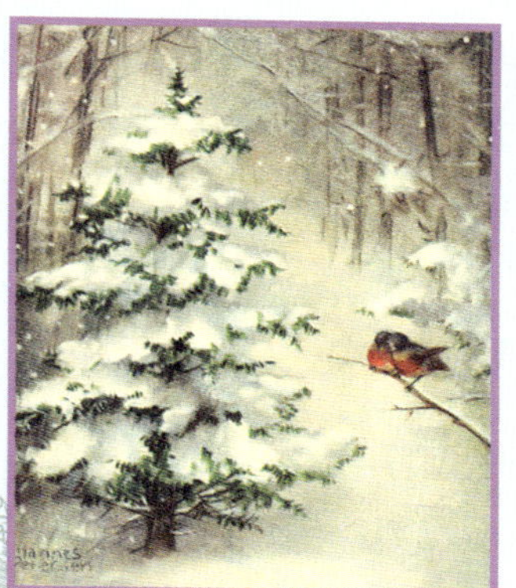

    The trial by market everything
        must come to.
I dallied so much with the
        thought of selling.
Then whether from mistaken
        courtesy
And fear of seeming short of
        speech, or whether
From hope of hearing good of
        what was mine,
I said, "There aren't enough to be
        worthwhile."

"I could soon tell how many they would cut,
You let me look them over."

"You could look.
But don't expect I'm going to let you have them."
Pasture they spring in, some in clumps too close
That lop each other of boughs, but not a few
Quite solitary and having equal boughs
All round and round. The latter he nodded "Yes" to,
Or paused to say beneath some lovelier one,
With a buyer's moderation, "That would do."
I thought so too, but wasn't there to say so.
We climbed the pasture on the south, crossed over,
And came down on the north.

He said, "A thousand."

"A thousand Christmas trees!—at what apiece?"

He felt some need of softening that to me:
"A thousand trees would come to thirty dollars."

Then I was certain I had never meant
To let him have them. Never show surprise!
But thirty dollars seemed so small beside
The extent of pasture I should strip, three cents
(For that was all they figured out apiece)—
Three cents so small beside the dollar friends
I should be writing to within the hour
Would pay in cities for good trees like those,
Regular vestry-trees whole Sunday Schools
Could hang enough on to pick off enough.

A thousand Christmas trees I didn't know I had!
Worth three cents more to give away than sell,
As may be shown by a simple calculation.
Too bad I couldn't lay one in a letter.
I can't help wishing I could send you one,
In wishing you herewith a Merry Christmas.

Good King Wenceslas

1. Good King Wenceslas look'd out
On the Feast of Stephen,
When the snow lay 'round about,
Deep and crisp and even.
Brightly shone the moon that night,
Tho' the forest was cruel,
When a poor man came in sight
Gath'ring winter fuel.

2. "Hither, page, and stand by me,
If thou know'st it, telling,
Yonder peasant, who is he?
Where and what his dwelling?"
"Sire, he lives a good league hence
Underneath the mountain;
Right against the forest fence,
By Saint Agnes fountain!"

3. "Bring me flesh, and bring me wine,
Bring me pinelogs hither;
Thou and I will see him dine
When we bear them hither."
Page and monarch forth they went,
Forth they went together:
Thro' the rude wind's wild lament
And the bitter weather.

4. "Sire, the night is darker now,
And the wind blows stronger;
Fails my heart, I know not how,
I can go no longer."
"Mark my footsteps, my good page.
Tread thou in them boldly,
Thou shalt find the winter's rage
Freeze thy blood less coldly!"

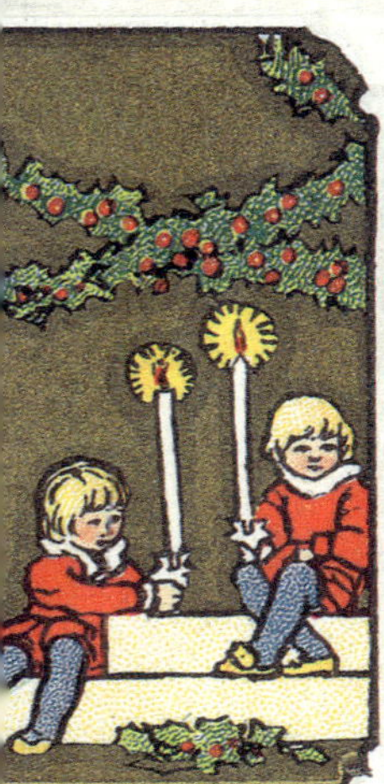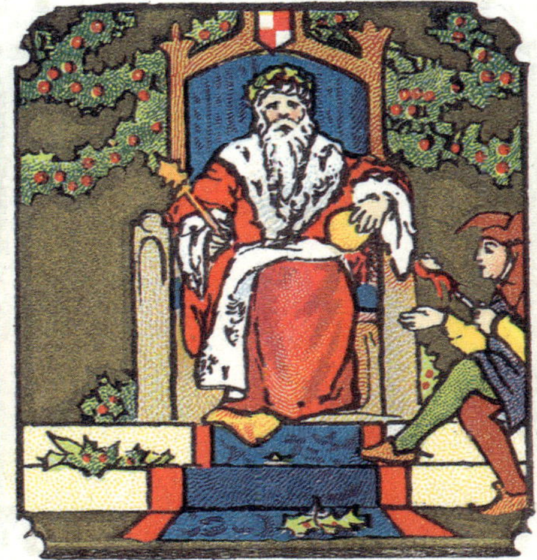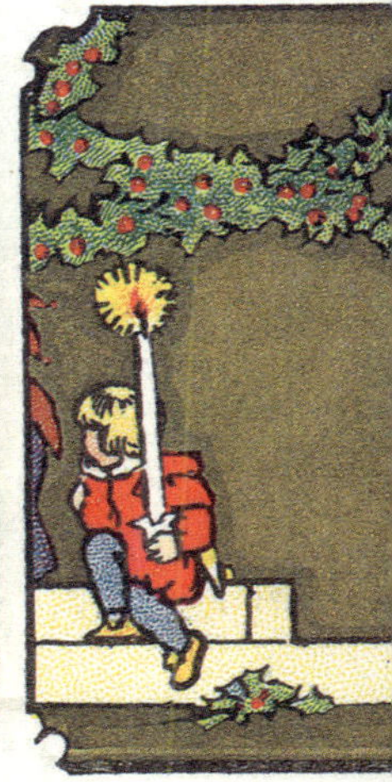

5. In his master's steps he trod,
Where the snow lay dinted;
Heat was in the very sod
Which the saint had printed;

Therefore, Christian men, be sure,
Wealth or rank possessing,
Ye who now will bless the poor,
Shall yourselves find blessing.

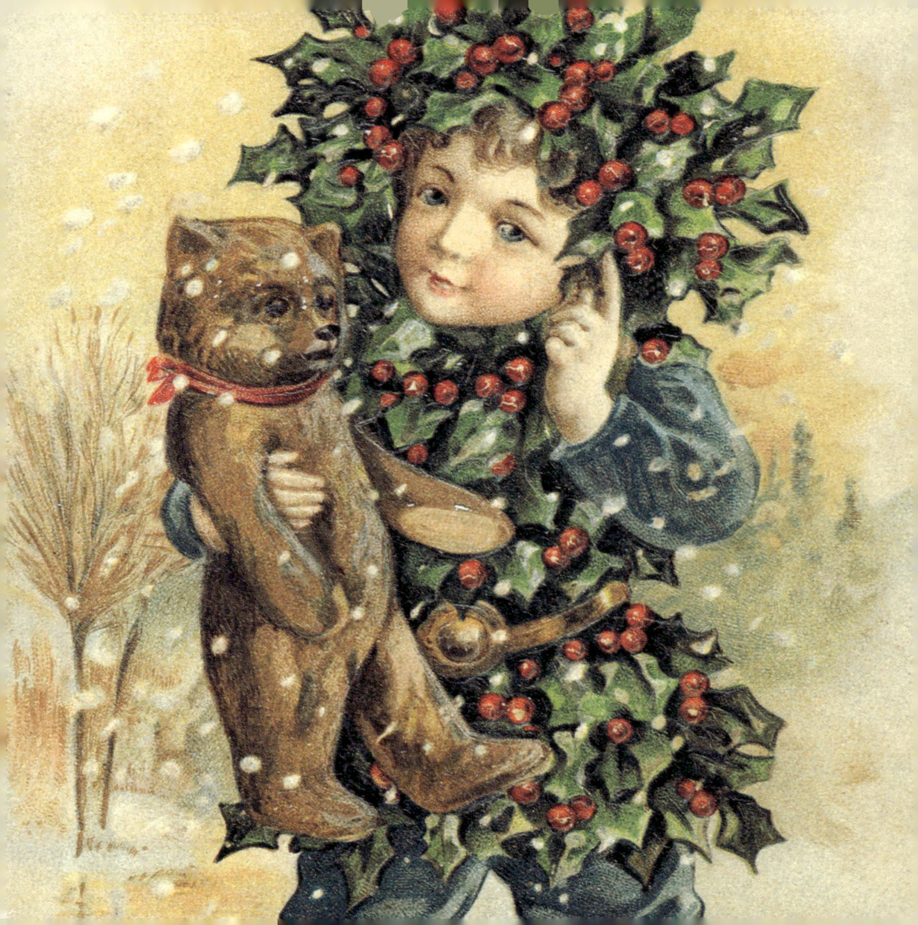

A Christmas Carol

MARTIN LUTHER

Ah! dearest Jesus. Holy Child.
Make Thee a bed, soft, undefil'd
Within my heart, that it may be
A quiet chamber kept for Thee.
My heart for very joy doth leap,
My lips no more can silence keep.
I too must sing, with joyful tongue.
That sweetest ancient cradle song.
    Glory to God in highest Heaven,
    Who unto man His Son hath
        given.
While angels sing, with pious mirth.
A glad New Year to all the earth.

The Twelve Days of Christmas

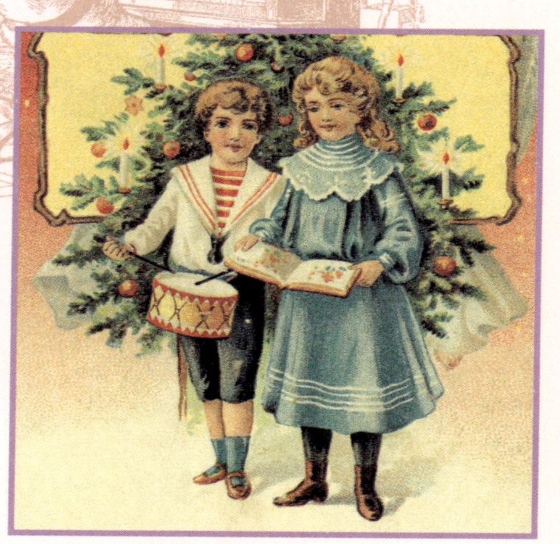

On the first day of Christmas my true love sent to me
A partridge in a pear tree.

On the second day of Christmas my true love sent to me
    Two turtle doves,
On the third day of Christmas my true love sent to me
    Three French hens,
On the fourth day of Christmas my true love sent to me
    Four mockingbirds,
On the fifth day of Christmas my true love sent to me
    Five golden rings,
On the sixth day of Christmas my true love sent to me
    Six geese a-laying,
On the seventh day of Christmas my true love sent to me
    Seven swans a-swimming,
On the eighth day of Christmas my true love sent to me
    Eight maids a-milking,
On the ninth day of Christmas my true love sent to me
    Nine ladies dancing,
On the tenth day of Christmas my true love sent to me
    Ten lords a-leaping,
On the eleventh day of Christmas my true love sent to me
    Eleven pipers piping,
On the twelfth day of Christmas my true love sent to me
    Twelve drummers drumming.

Holly Song

from *As You Like It*
WILLIAM SHAKESPEARE

Blow blow thou winter winde,
Thou art not so unkinde,
  As man's ingratitude
Thy tooth is not so keene,
Because thou art not seene,
  Although thy breath be rude.
Heigh ho, sing heigh ho, unto the
  greene holly.
Most friendship, is fayning; most
  Loving, meere folly;
Then heigh ho, the holly.
  This Life is most jolly.

Freize, freize, thou bitter skie
Thou dost not bight so nigh
  As benefitts forgot;
Though thou the waters warpe,
Thy sting is not so sharpe,
  As friend remembered not,
Heigh ho, sing heigh ho, unto the
  greene holly,
Most friendship, is faying; most
  Loving, meere folly;
Then heigh ho, the holly,
This Life is most jolly.

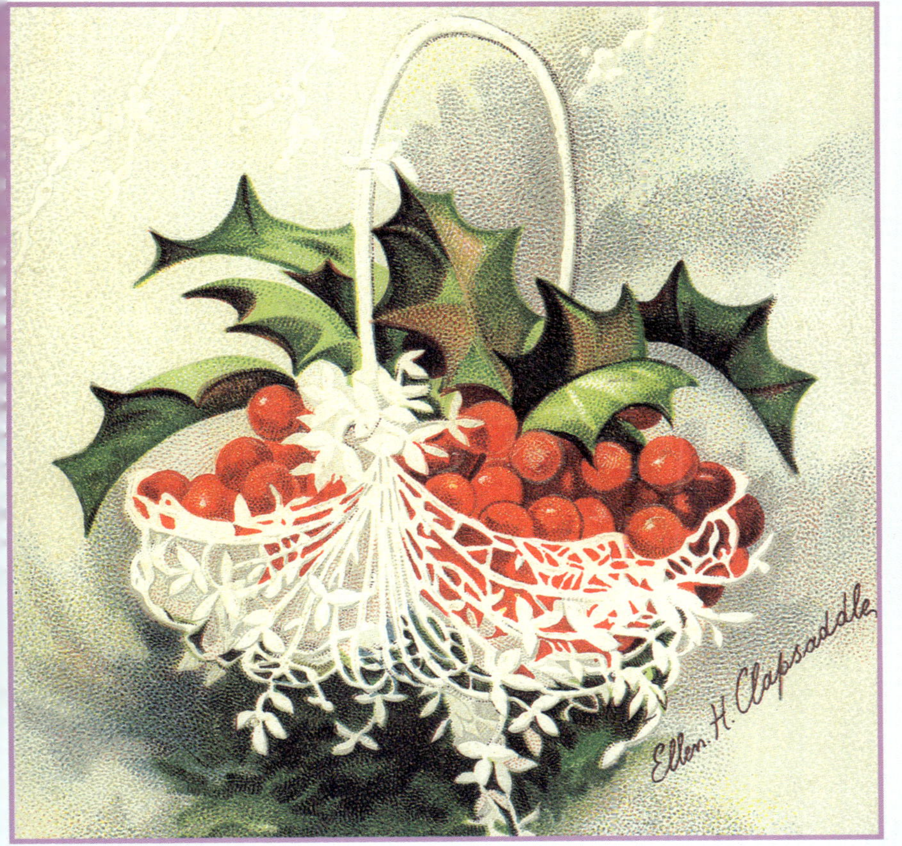
Ellen. H. Clapsaddle.

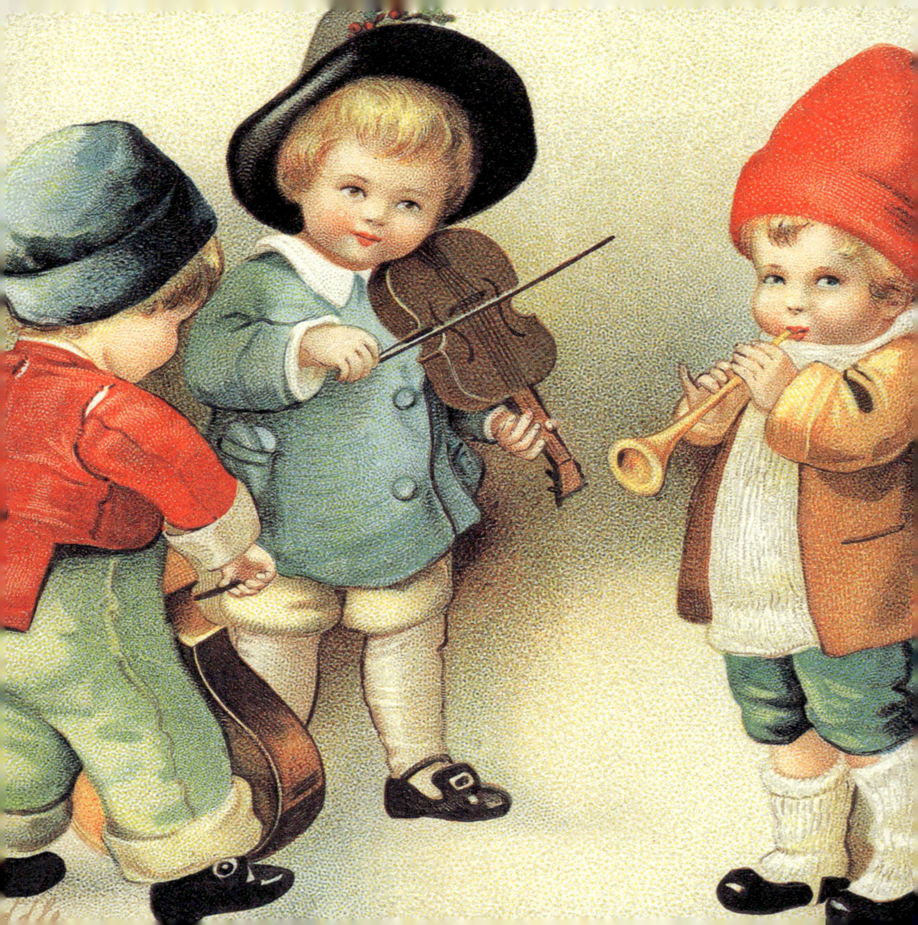

Joy to the World!

1. Joy to the world! The Lord is come;
Let earth receive her King.
Let every heart prepare Him room,
And heaven and nature sing,
And heaven and nature sing,
And heaven and heaven and nature sing.

2. Joy to the world! The Saviour reigns;
Let men their songs employ;
While fields and floods, rocks, hills and plains
Repeat the sounding joy,
Repeat the sounding joy,
Repeat, repeat the sounding joy.

3. He rules the world with truth and grace,
And makes the nations prove
The glories of His righteousness,
And wonders of His love,
And wonders of His love,
And wonders, and wonders of
    His Love.

Mistletoe

Walter de la Mare

Sitting under the mistletoe
(Pale-green, fairy mistletoe),
One last candle burning low,
All the sleepy dancers gone,
Just one candle burning on,
Shadows lurking everywhere:
Some one came, and kissed me there.

Tired I was; my head would go
Nodding under the mistletoe
(Pale-green, fairy mistletoe),
No footsteps came, no voice, but only,
Just as I sat there, sleepy, lonely,
Stooped in the still and shadowy air
Lips unseen——and kissed me there.

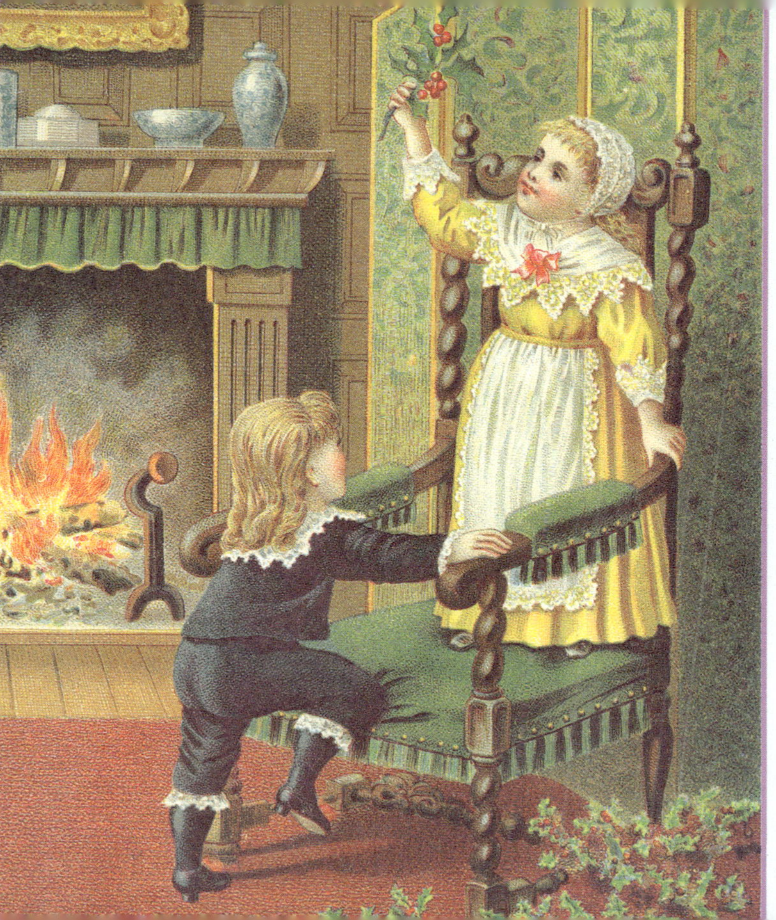

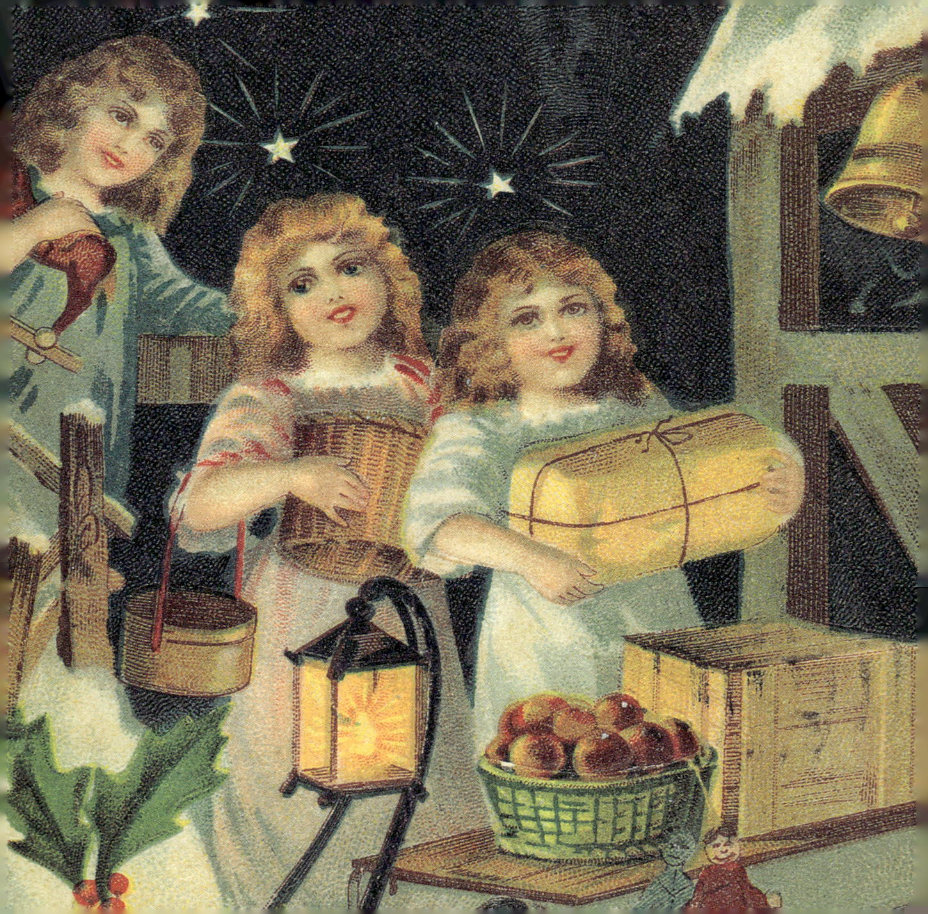

Into the Darkest Hour

MADELEINE L'ENGLE

It was a time like this
was and tumult of war,
a horror in the air.
Hungry yawned the abyss—
and yet there came the star
and the child most wonderfully there.

It was a time like this
of fear & lust for power,
license & greed & blight—
and yet the Prince of bliss
came in the darkest hour
in quiet & silent light.

And in a time like this
how celebrate his birth
when all things fall apart?
Ah! wonderful it is
with no room on the earth
the stable is our heart.

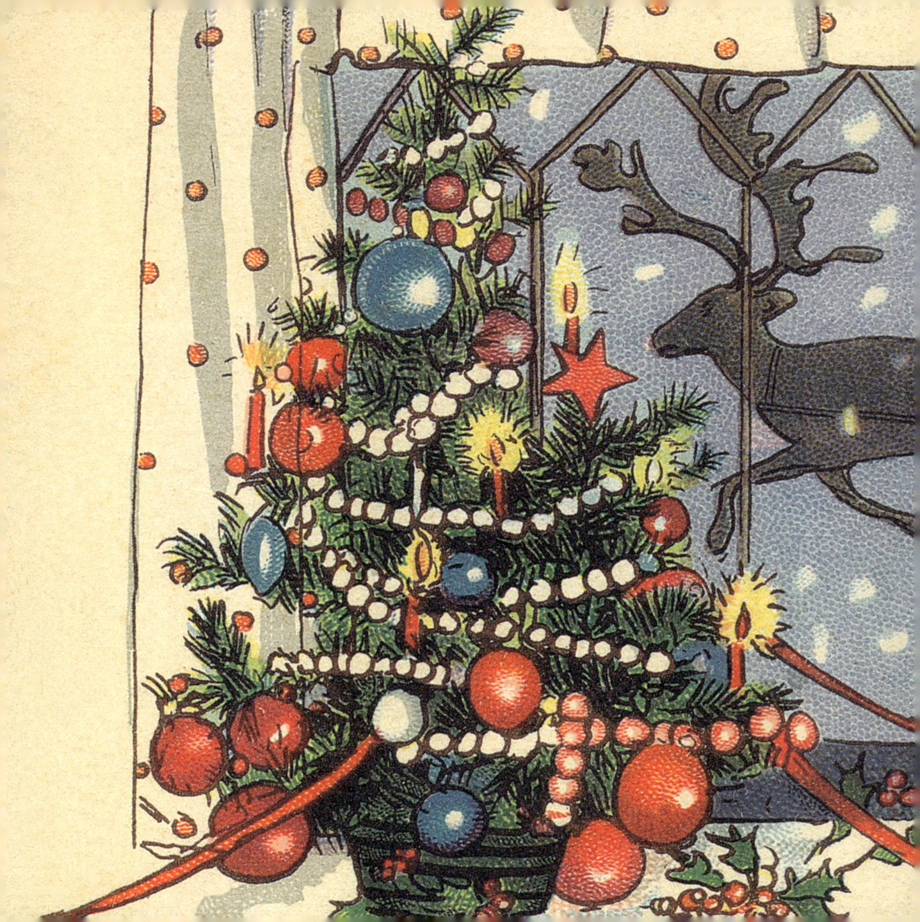

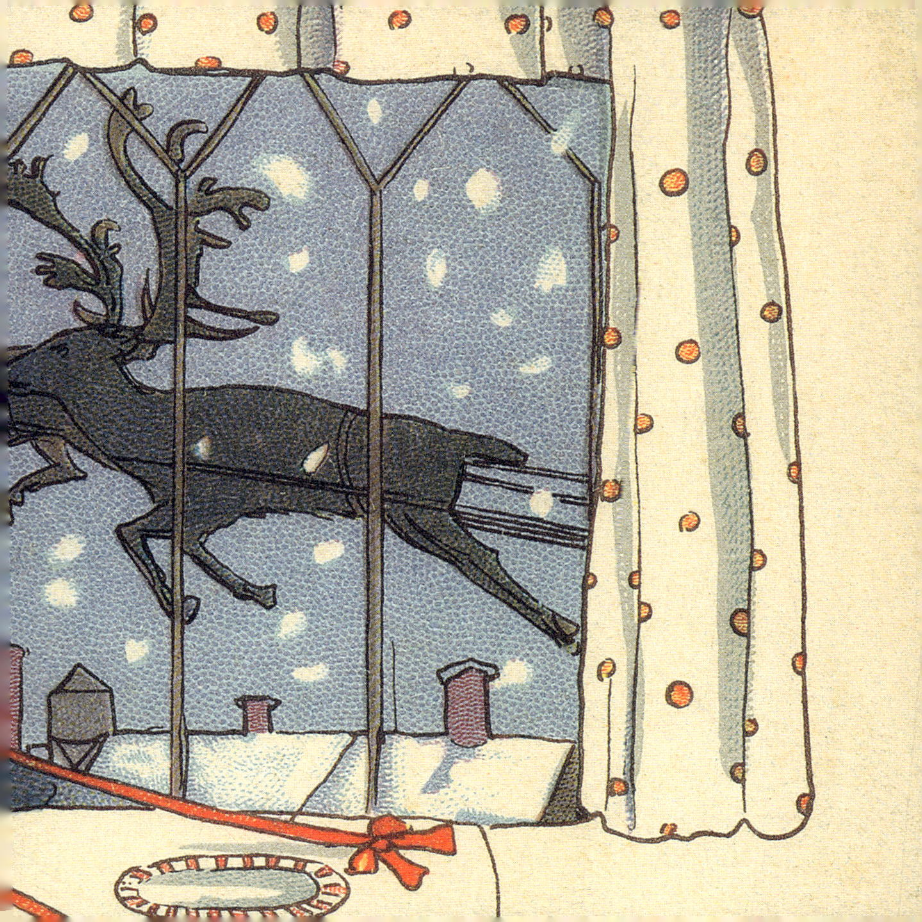

Voices in the Mist

ALFRED TENNYSON

The time draws near the birth of
　　Christ.
　The moon is hid, the night is still.
　The Christmas bells from hill to hill
Answer each other in the mist.

Four voices of four hamlets round,
　From far and near, on mead and
　　　moor,
　Swell out and fail, as if a door
Were shut before me and the sound:

Each voice four changes on the wind,
　That now dilate, and note decrease,
　Peace and goodwill, goodwill and
　　peace,
Peace and goodwill, to all mankind.

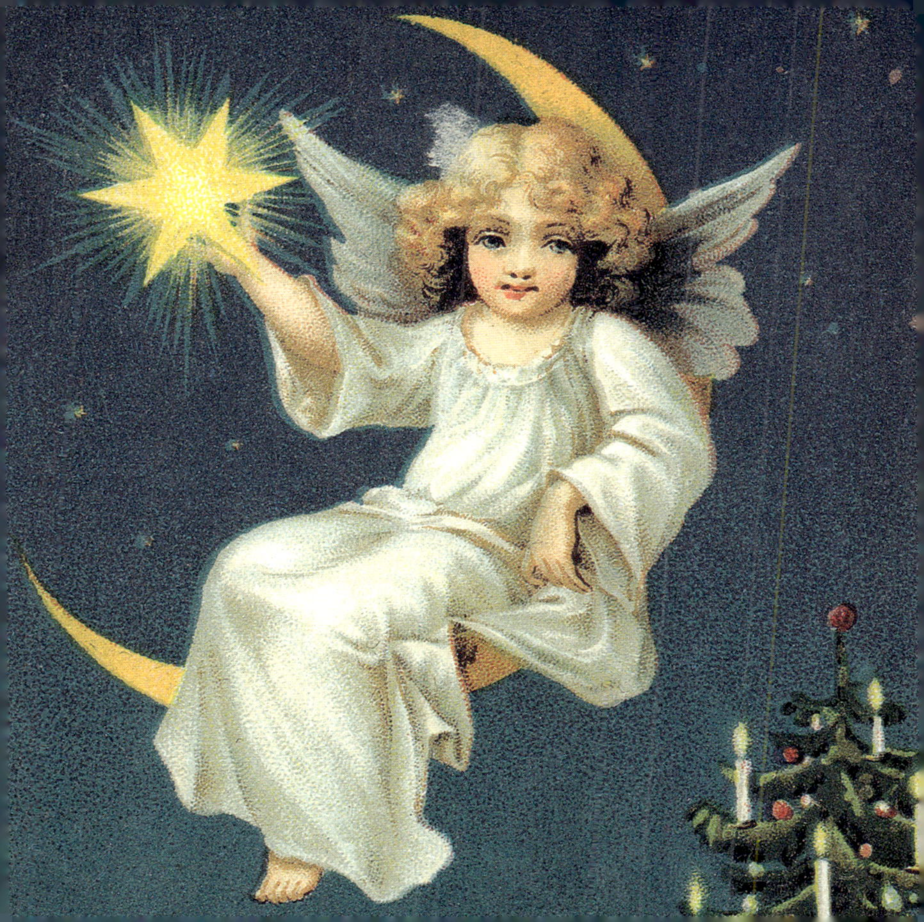

Frosty the Snowman

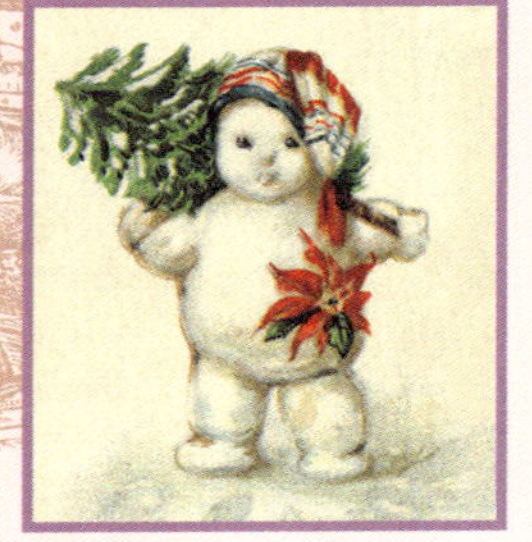

Frosty the Snowman, was a jolly happy soul,
With a corncob pipe and a button nose, and two eyes made out of coal.
Frosty the Snowman, is a fairy tale they say.
He was made of snow, but the children know how he came to life one day.

There must have been some magic in that old silk hat they found,
For when they placed it on his head he began to dance around!

Oh, Frosty the Snowman was alive as he could be;
And the children say he could laugh and play,
Just the same as you and me.

Thumpety thump, thump, thumpety thump, thump
Look at Frosty go
Thumpety thump, thump, thumpety thump, thump
Over the hills of snow.

Frosty the Snowman, knew the sun was hot that day,
So he said "Let's run, and we'll have some fun now, before I melt away."

Down to the village, with a broomstick in his hand,
Running here and there, all around the square,
Saying, "Catch me if you can."

He led them down the streets of town, right to the traffic cop;
And only paused a moment, when he heard him holler, "Stop!"

For Frosty, the Snowman, had to hurry on his way,
But he waved goodbye, saying "Don't you cry, I'll be back again some day."

Thumpety thump, thump, thumpety thump, thump
Look at Frosty go.
Thumpety thump, thump, thumpety thump, thump
Over hills of snow.

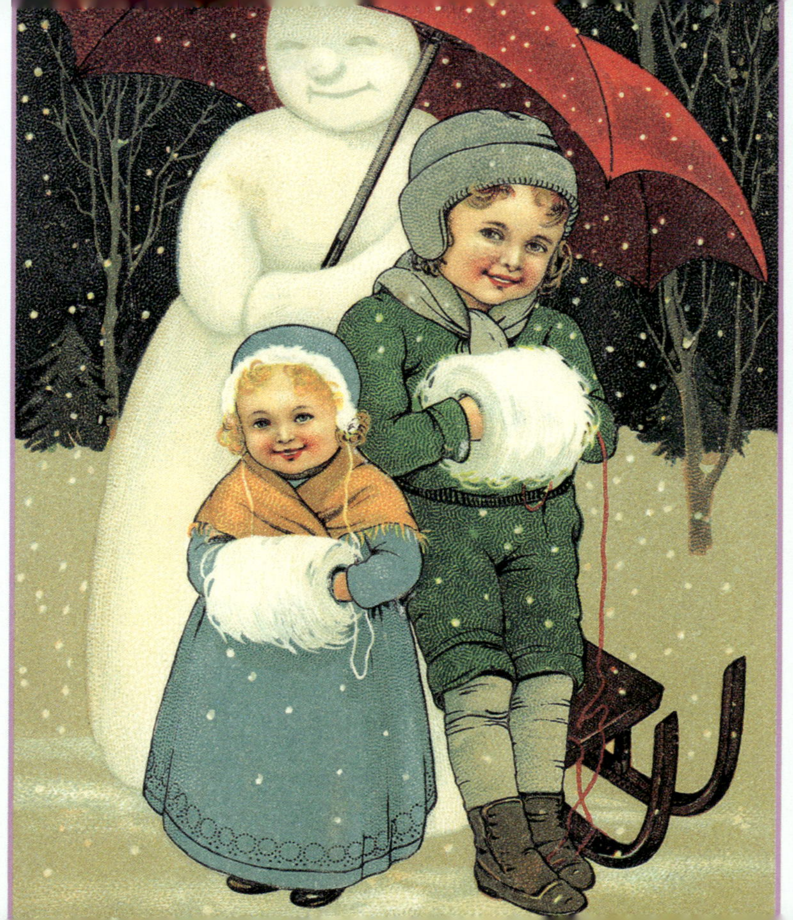

Let Us Keep Christmas

GRACE NOLL CROWELL

Whatever else be lost among the years,
Let us keep Christmas still a shining thing:
Whatever doubts assail us, or what fears,
Let us hold close one day, remembering
Its poignant meaning for the hearts of men.
Let us get back our childlike faith again.

Well, So That Is That

W. H. Auden

Well, so that is that. Now we must dismantle the tree,
Putting the decorations back into their cardboard boxes—
Some have got broken—and carrying them up to the attic.
The holly and mistletoe must be taken down and burnt,
And the children got ready for school. There are enough
Left-overs to do, warmed up, for the rest of the week—
Not that we have much appetite, having drunk such a lot,
Stayed up so late, attempted—quite unsuccessfully—
To love all our relatives, and in general
Grossly overestimated our powers. Once again
As in previous years we have seen the actual Vision and failed
To do more than entertain it as an agreeable
Possibility, once again we have sent Him away
Begging though to remain His disobedient servant,
The promising child who cannot keep His word for long.

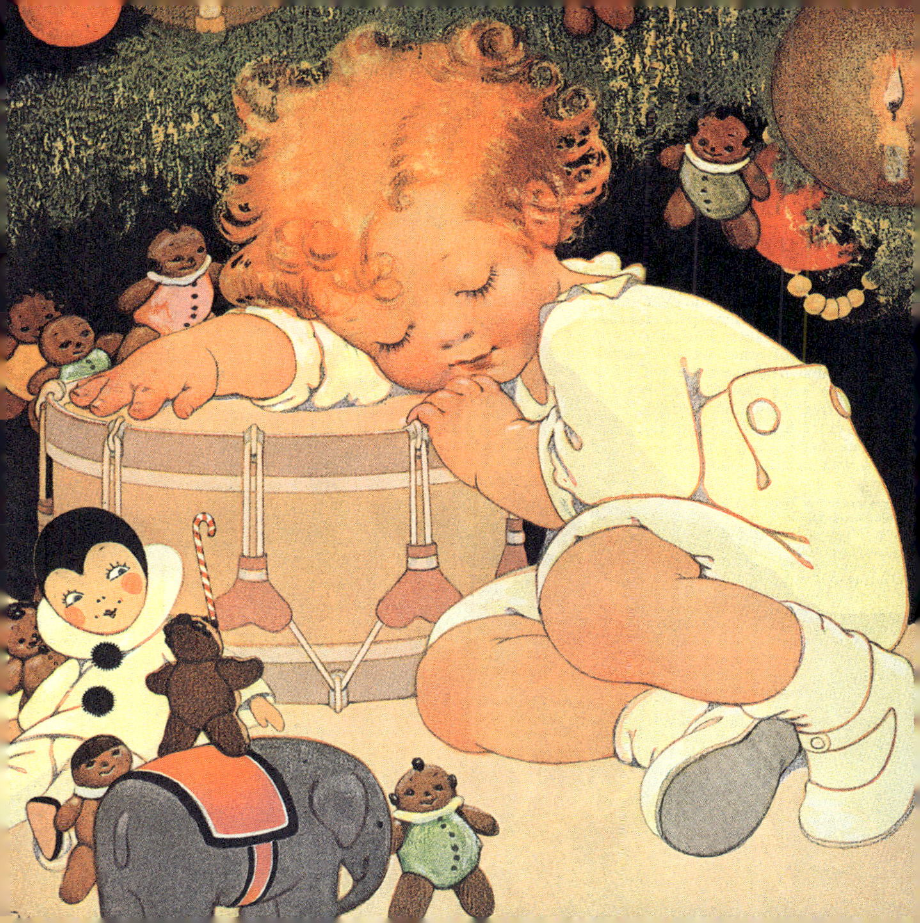

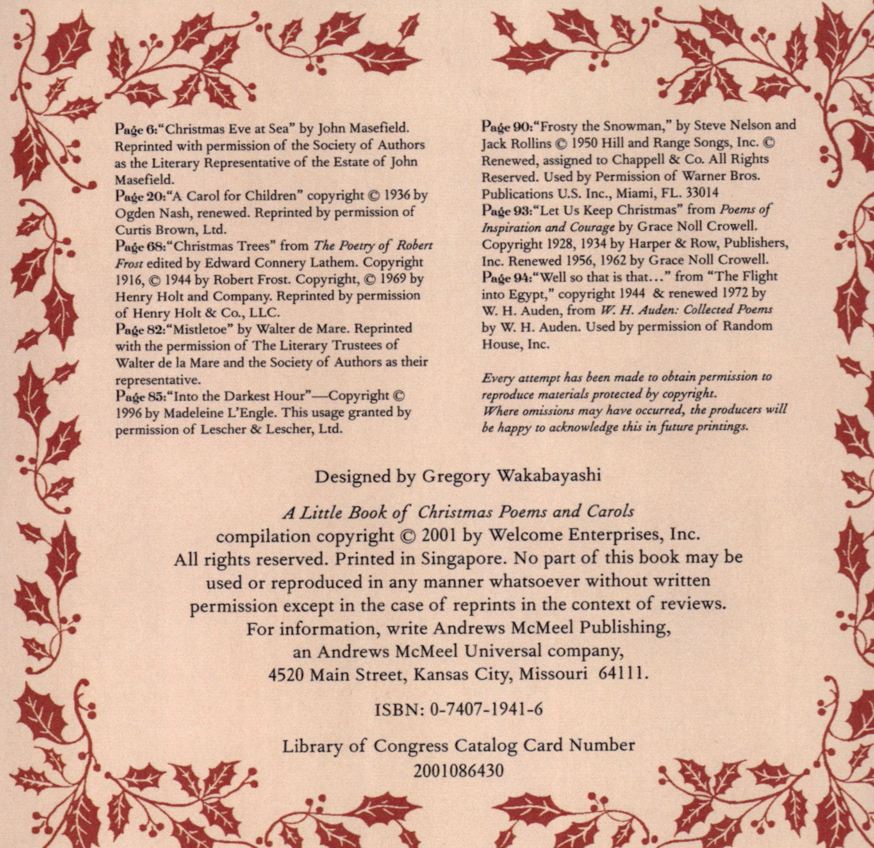

Page 6: "Christmas Eve at Sea" by John Masefield. Reprinted with permission of the Society of Authors as the Literary Representative of the Estate of John Masefield.

Page 20: "A Carol for Children" copyright © 1936 by Ogden Nash, renewed. Reprinted by permission of Curtis Brown, Ltd.

Page 68: "Christmas Trees" from *The Poetry of Robert Frost* edited by Edward Connery Lathem. Copyright 1916, © 1944 by Robert Frost. Copyright, © 1969 by Henry Holt and Company. Reprinted by permission of Henry Holt & Co., LLC.

Page 82: "Mistletoe" by Walter de Mare. Reprinted with the permission of The Literary Trustees of Walter de la Mare and the Society of Authors as their representative.

Page 85: "Into the Darkest Hour"—Copyright © 1996 by Madeleine L'Engle. This usage granted by permission of Lescher & Lescher, Ltd.

Page 90: "Frosty the Snowman," by Steve Nelson and Jack Rollins © 1950 Hill and Range Songs, Inc. © Renewed, assigned to Chappell & Co. All Rights Reserved. Used by Permission of Warner Bros. Publications U.S. Inc., Miami, FL. 33014

Page 93: "Let Us Keep Christmas" from *Poems of Inspiration and Courage* by Grace Noll Crowell. Copyright 1928, 1934 by Harper & Row, Publishers, Inc. Renewed 1956, 1962 by Grace Noll Crowell.

Page 94: "Well so that is that…" from "The Flight into Egypt," copyright 1944 & renewed 1972 by W. H. Auden, from *W. H. Auden: Collected Poems* by W. H. Auden. Used by permission of Random House, Inc.

Every attempt has been made to obtain permission to reproduce materials protected by copyright. Where omissions may have occurred, the producers will be happy to acknowledge this in future printings.

Designed by Gregory Wakabayashi